Introduction to Adaptive Trial Designs and Protocols

Introduction to Adaptive Trial Designs and Master Protocols

Jay J. H. Park
McMaster University, Ontario

Edward J. Mills
McMaster University, Ontario

J. Kyle Wathen
Cytel, Cambridge, Massachusetts

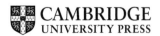
CAMBRIDGE
UNIVERSITY PRESS

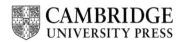

Shaftesbury Road, Cambridge CB2 8EA, United Kingdom

One Liberty Plaza, 20th Floor, New York, NY 10006, USA

477 Williamstown Road, Port Melbourne, VIC 3207, Australia

314–321, 3rd Floor, Plot 3, Splendor Forum, Jasola District Centre, New Delhi – 110025, India

103 Penang Road, #05–06/07, Visioncrest Commercial, Singapore 238467

Cambridge University Press is part of Cambridge University Press & Assessment, a department of the University of Cambridge.

We share the University's mission to contribute to society through the pursuit of education, learning and research at the highest international levels of excellence.

www.cambridge.org
Information on this title: www.cambridge.org/9781108926980

DOI: 10.1017/9781108917919

First published 2023

Printed in the United Kingdom by CPI Group Ltd, Croydon CR0 4YY

A catalogue record for this publication is available from the British Library.

ISBN 978-1-108-92698-0 Paperback

Cambridge University Press & Assessment has no responsibility for the persistence or accuracy of URLs for external or third-party internet websites referred to in this publication and does not guarantee that any content on such websites is, or will remain, accurate or appropriate.

....

Every effort has been made in preparing this book to provide accurate and up-to-date information that is in accord with accepted standards and practice at the time of publication. Although case histories are drawn from actual cases, every effort has been made to disguise the identities of the individuals involved. Nevertheless, the authors, editors, and publishers can make no warranties that the information contained herein is totally free from error, not least because clinical standards are constantly changing through research and regulation. The authors, editors, and publishers therefore disclaim all liability for direct or consequential damages resulting from the use of material contained in this book. Readers are strongly advised to pay careful attention to information provided by the manufacturer of any drugs or equipment that they plan to use.

Content

Preface

When we think of clinical trials, we mostly imagine 'one shot' two-arm trials. These conventional trials evaluating a single intervention against placebo or some standard-of-care as a control group are designed with a fixed sample size that is predetermined at the design stage based on a variety of assumptions, and the statistical analysis occurs once after the recruitment reaches this predetermined target. There are other approaches to clinical trials that can broadly be classified into two methods of 'adaptive trial designs' and 'master protocols'.

Adaptive trial designs refer to a type of design that allows for pre-specified modifications to trial designs during the trial in response to accumulated trial data. For many research questions, by being able to respond to the trial data mid-trial, adaptive trial design can have important efficiencies over fixed sample trial designs. *Master protocols* refer to a single overarching protocol designed to answer multiple interventional questions. The framework of master protocols aims to create a common trial infrastructure in which multiple interventions can be evaluated using the standardised rules that are outlined in the protocol. Instead of two-arm conventional trials, the master protocol framework aims to reduce the need for redundant clinical trials and enable multiple interventions and hypotheses to be tested by bringing a collaborative approach to clinical trial research.

In this book, we hope to assist investigators to gain confidence and a clear understanding of adaptive trial designs and master protocols. This book is intended for those with minimal background in clinical trial research and to help readers grasp strengths and limitations of these novel designs and apply them to their own areas of research and clinical practice. For those who plan to conduct clinical trial research over a long period of time, this book is intended to be read before tackling other technically oriented books or papers for further methodological development and implementation.

Introduction to Adaptive Trial Designs and Master Protocols is divided into five parts. In *Part I*, we define the concepts of clinical research, clinical trial phases, and randomisation and summarise conventional approaches to clinical trials research. The concept of exploratory research (hypothesis-generating research) and confirmatory research (hypothesis-confirming research) is discussed, since the appropriateness of a specific research design depends on the type of research question that is being asked. Before more detailed discussion of adaptive trial designs and master protocols occurs, it is important that the reader gain an understanding of concepts including p-values, statistical power, and other relevant concepts in frequentist and Bayesian statistics. An overview is given in the first chapter to help bridge the gap for readers less familiar with any of these topics.

Part II introduces the reader to the basic ingredients of adaptive trial designs. Before having a more elaborative discussion of how adaptive trial designs in trials being conducted under the master protocol framework, it is important to understand the principles of adaptive trial designs and their common types. As more planning is required in adaptive trial designs relative to traditional trial designs through extensive clinical trial simulations, it is important for the reader to understand how simulations work and are used to come up with decision rules and other features of adaptive clinical trials.

In *Part III*, the key attributes of the concept of master protocols and their sub-categories (basket trials, umbrella trials, and platform trials) are introduced and differentiated from adaptive trial designs for the reader. Some master protocol trials may be designed with fixed sample designs, so it is important to distinguish the concept of master protocols from adaptive trial designs. Basket trials and umbrella trials are compared and contrasted, as students often mistake one for the other. Adaptive platform randomised trials, also known as multi-arm, multi-stage designs, are introduced and compared to other types of adaptive trial designs.

Part IV is intended to improve the reader's ability to comprehend and critically appraise published results of clinical trials that are designed using adaptive trial designs and master protocols. Thus, this section is dedicated to the discussion of published case studies of adaptive clinical trials, basket trials, umbrella trials, and platform trials. In this section, general guidelines on what to look for when reading results or a proposal of adaptive clinical trials and master protocols is provided as well as specific guidelines for common types of adaptive trial designs and master protocols.

Part V introduces the reader to common misconceptions and practical considerations for adaptive trial designs and master protocols. Common misconceptions about adaptive trial designs and master protocols are discussed here to differentiate and clarify the issues that are specific to these novel designs as opposed to those that apply to any clinical research. The practical considerations regarding funding and implementation of clinical trials using adaptive trial designs and master protocol frameworks are drawn from the authors' personal professional experience.

Each chapter is written to be as self-contained as possible. There are introductory summaries of the chapter mission statement and chapter goals. Where applicable, there are three to five bullet point summaries of the material provided in each chapter.

About the Authors

Jay J. H. Park is a trained Clinical Trialist with expertise in adaptive trial designs and master protocols. He holds a faculty position in the Department of Health Research Methods, Evidence, and Impact within the Faculty of Health Sciences at McMaster University. At McMaster University, he teaches HRM 732, the first available graduate-level course on adaptive clinical trial design and master protocols.

Edward Mills is a trained Clinical Trialist and a faculty member who co-teaches HRM 732 at McMaster University. He has founded several consulting companies that have specialised in Bayesian evidence synthesis, highly efficient clinical trials, and platform trials.

J. Kyle Wathen is a trained Bayesian Statistician with over 20 years of experience in statistical research and development of software and simulation-guided designs for drug development. He is the Vice Chair of the Statistical Software Working Group for the biopharmaceutical section of the American Statistical Association. Vice President of Scientific Strategy and Innovation at Cytel Inc. He has been involved in the scientific design and simulation of many platform trials and has over 10 years of experience in this area.

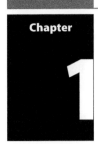

Introduction to Clinical Trial Research

Jay J. H. Park, J. Kyle Wathen, and Edward J. Mills

Key Points of This Chapter

This chapter introduces clinical research concepts and randomised clinical trials, covering the basics and building blocks that are necessary to understand the topics of adaptive trial designs and master protocols.

The key points of this chapter are:

- Clinical trials are a type of prospective experimental study in which human volunteers receive specific interventions according to the research protocol; then they are followed longitudinally over time. Clinical trials are typically conducted in a series of sequence (from phase I, phase IIA, phase IIB, and phase III) that builds on knowledge accumulated from non-clinical and previous clinical studies.

- Randomisation is a process of random assignment of clinical trial participants to one or more intervention group(s) or control group under comparison. The use of randomisation provides a sound basis for making statistical causal inference when estimating the comparative treatment effects between groups. Randomisation removes selection bias and tends to produce groups that are on average comparable in terms of both observable and unobservable factors.

- Equipoise, a genuine state of uncertainty or conflict about relative merits of a set of competing interventions, provides justification of randomised clinical trials and speaks to ethical acceptability of randomisation.

- Fixed sample trial design refers to a type of design in which the trial data are only analysed once, when a priori determined sample size has been reached. Fixed sample trial designs are designed with a fixed maximum sample size, a fixed number of interventions, and a defined end to the trial. This is the most common approach to clinical trial research.

Clinical Research Basics

Clinical Trials and Observational Studies

Clinical research, a type of medical research, uses human volunteers. The terminologies of clinical research and clinical trials are often used interchangeability, with some researchers often using a narrow definition of clinical research as being clinical trials. Clinical research can be broadly classified into two main types of clinical studies: *clinical trials* (also referred to as interventional studies) and *observational studies* [1].

1

There are several important differences between clinical trials and observational studies. Clinical trials are a type of prospective experimental or interventional studies in which human volunteers (also commonly referred to as participants or patients) receive specific interventions according to the research protocol then followed longitudinally over time. The main goal of clinical trial research is to advance scientific knowledge while minimising risks for the individual participants. Clinical trials are experiments. Given the experimental nature of clinical trial research, participation in clinical trials is not without potential risk.

In observational studies, investigators 'observe' individuals without assigning them to any specific intervention(s). There are observational studies, such as cross-sectional studies, that only describe disease status, exposure, and other characteristics of human participants at a given point in time. Even in longitudinal observational studies that describe participants over time, some are retrospective in nature in which human subjects may be identified retrospectively from electronic health records or other existing data sources.

In this book, we will use the broad definition of interventions as any manipulation of the participant and/or their environment for the purpose of improving their health outcome(s). A large proportion of interventions that end up being evaluated in clinical trial research involve therapeutic biomedical interventions, such as drugs and biologics, but other types of interventions such as medical devices, vaccines, procedures, and education can also be evaluated using clinical trials. Observational studies often may only consider a risk factor, such as smoking status, for their research question. Human participants of observational studies are not assigned to specific interventions according to the protocol developed by the investigators. Participants can receive medical interventions, but these are part of their routine medical care. Interventions in clinical trials that are provided to participants can be heavily standardised, as outlined in the trial protocol.

While not all clinical trials use randomisation to assign patients to specific intervention(s), the use of randomisation is another key difference between observational studies to randomised clinical trials. In randomised clinical trials, commonly shorten to RCTs, the collective data of each interventional group are compared against each other or against the control group to determine the comparative efficacy of the experimental intervention group [1]. In non-randomised clinical trials, there is no random assignment of the intervention(s), but they are still prospective and interventional in nature. Non-randomised clinical trials can be conducted as single-arm clinical trials, without a control group, or as two or more arms.

Clinical Trial Phases

Clinical trials are conducted in a sequence that builds on knowledge accumulated from previous clinical and non-clinical studies. While the actual sequence of clinical trials conducted may vary, clinical trial sequence is often described as four phases (phase I to phase III) where information from early phase studies is used to support and plan later phase studies.

In phase I of a clinical trial, the focus is on the safety of a drug. Phase I of a trial generally involves healthy volunteers or patients who have the condition or the disease for which the drug is intended. The objectives of phase I studies are to determine the initial safety and tolerability of the dose range that is expected to be evaluated in later phase studies and also to characterise the pharmacokinetics (how the body absorbs the drug) and pharmaco-dynamics (how the body reacts to a drug). Phase I studies are usually conducted after promising findings are demonstrated from in vitro, animal model, and other pre-clinical research studies, so they are often instances during which an investigational product is first administered to humans.

After the safety, dose range, and clinical pharmacology are determined from initial phase I studies, phase II studies (also referred to as exploratory studies) are conducted. A phase II of a clinical trial is designed to investigate safety and efficacy in the target population for which the drug is intended. Broad goals of phase II studies are to demonstrate proof-of-efficacy, to better characterise the dose-response relationship of the experimental therapies, and to evaluate whether these therapies have any biological activity or clinical effect to determine whether a large phase III study is warranted. Phase II studies typically include multiple trials conducted in different stages, often called phase IIA and phase IIB. Phase IIA studies are often referred to as proof-of-concept studies that are usually conducted to demonstrate clinical signals with a small number of patients [2]. If the phase IIA study provides proof-of-efficacy, a phase IIB study is often conducted on a larger number of patients to determine the optimal dose(s) for the subsequent phase III confirmatory trials [2]. As there is often uncertainty in dose-response relationship of experimental therapies, both types of phase II studies may investigate multiple doses.

Phase III studies, also known as confirmatory or pivotal studies, are conducted to confirm whether an experimental therapy offers a clinical benefit to a specific population and to examine its safety profile. Phase III studies are most often randomised clinical trials that compare one or more new interventions against the control group to demonstrate whether the experimental intervention(s) can offer clinical benefits. The choice in the control group may include a placebo or a current standard-of-care treatment, should an existing treatment be available in the target population. Evidence from phase III studies is often required to obtain approval from regulatory bodies such as the U.S. Food and Drug Administration. Phase III studies are considerably larger than earlier phase studies and longer in duration, so they can provide more informative long-term or rare side effects of the experimental therapy.

Early phase studies such as phase I and IIA may be conducted as non-randomised or single-arm clinical trials and rarely have a control group. Phase IIB studies are often conducted as a randomised study with a concurrent control group to further explore efficacy and safety of candidate therapies and to define the optimal dosing regimen that will be subsequently tested in a phase III trial. A concurrent control group consists of subjects who were concurrently enrolled from the same study population and followed under the same protocol as the subjects who were randomly assigned into the treatment group(s) [3]. In non-randomised trials, a historical control group that comes from different study populations may be used as performance criteria to determine whether subsequent clinical trials are warranted for further clinical trial investigation [4]. For instance, a non-randomised phase IIA trial may deem that a given experimental therapy is warranted for further clinical trial investigation in a phase IIB study, if the rate of favourable clinical response observed at the end of the study exceeds a pre-specified criterion that may be determined from a response rate from historical control group.

Randomisation

Randomisation refers to a process of randomly assigning clinical trial participants to one or more experimental intervention group(s) or control group under comparison [5, 6]. Many consider randomised clinical trials to be the most valid method for establishing efficacy and safety of medical interventions. Randomisation removes selection bias and provides a sound statistical basis for establishing causality [7]. Unbiased allocation through properly conducted randomisation can help ascribe the observed difference in clinical outcomes as treatment effects to the interventions that are being compared in a given clinical trial [1, 7]. Randomisation, on average, tends to produce groups that are comparable in terms of both measurable and unmeasurable factors [6]. Randomisation does not guarantee balance between groups being evaluated, but balance of baseline prognostic factors is not necessary for valid causal inference [8, 9]. Even with randomisation, imbalances can occur by random chance rather than as a result of some systematic bias [10].

Randomisation Techniques

Simple randomisation is a type of unrestricted randomisation in which the randomisation is solely based on a single constant allocation ratio. A simple randomisation in a two-arm trial at equal allocation (1:1) is equivalent to tossing a coin to determine each assignment [5, 6]. With a typical coin, there is equal probability of the coin flip landing as a head or a tail. In a series of coin tosses, obtaining consecutive heads or tails is not unlikely [6]. If you flipped the coin 10 times consecutively, it is not unlikely that the number of times the coin landed on heads would be different from the number of times it landed on tails. As in the case of the coin toss scenario, the use of simple randomisation may result in imbalance in sample size with a long series of assignments favouring one group over the other group, especially when the sample size is relatively small [11]. While the probability of imbalance will generally decrease as the sample size increases, simple randomisation is not often used in modern clinical trials [12].

Instead of simple randomisation, other randomisation techniques such as block randomisation and stratified randomisation are often used [11, 12]. Block randomisation is a type of restricted randomisation method that helps balance the number of patients assigned to each group [6, 11]. Block randomisation can help maximise statistical power by assigning equal numbers of patients between study groups. The randomisation scheme consists of a sequence of blocks that contains a pre-specified number of assignments in a random order, such that patient allocations are balanced in terms of the desired allocation ratio. In a two-arm trial with block randomisation at an equal allocation ratio, the number of patients randomised to the treatment and control would be split in half within each block size. For example, within a block size of four, two patients would be assigned to the control and the other two patients to the treatment group in a random order (e.g., AABB, ABAB, ABBA, BAAB, BABA, and BBAA). There is a potential concern of bias with block randomisation if the treatment assignments become known or predictable [11, 13]. With a block size of four, if the investigator knew the assignment of first three patients in the block, the next assignment is no longer concealed. Lack of allocation concealment can lead to selection bias. To minimise concerns for selection bias, random block sizes that are reasonably large and blinding procedures are often used with block randomisation.

Stratified randomisation is a type of restricted randomisation method that is used to balance one or a few pre-specified prognostic factors between groups [11, 14]. One or more prognostic characteristics that are measurable at baseline can be used to define strata in which patients are separately randomised. For instance, if randomisation was stratified by sex (male vs. female), there would be two separate randomisation schemes generated, where male participants would be separately randomised from female participants. If randomisation was stratified by sex with two levels and another prognostic factor of disease severity with three levels (mild vs. moderate vs. severe) on top of sex, this would create a total of 6 strata ($2 \times 3 = 6$). Stratified randomisation can help balance between treatment groups with respect to pre-specified prognostic factor(s), as long as there is sufficient sample size in each stratum, so it is important to keep the number of strata at a minimum [11, 15]. When there are too many prognostic factors that end up being used for stratified randomisation, this can result in too many strata being created and some of the strata would then be sparse or be empty. The use of simple randomisation within each strata is equivalent to simple randomisation without stratification [16]. For instance, flipping multiple coins within strata is equivalent to just flipping a coin. The use of stratified randomisation requires a restricted randomisation, such as block randomisation, to ensure a degree of balance within strata, so it is often the case that 'stratified block randomisation' is used in clinical trials [11].

Equipoise

Equipoise refers to a state of genuine uncertainty or conflict about relative merits of a set of interventions [17]. Personal equipoise exists when an individual clinician has no preference or is uncertain about the relative merits of the interventions [18]. Clinical equipoise, on the other hand, refers to a state in which there is uncertainty or conflicting expert opinions about a set of interventions [18]. The conflicting role of personal versus clinical equipoise in clinical trial research is a common misunderstanding. Even when personal equipoise may not exist for the treating clinician, clinical equipoise can exist in a set of interventions included in a clinical trial [18].

The principle of clinical equipoise provides justification of randomised clinical trials and ethical acceptability of being randomly allocated to an intervention group or a control group [17]. The goal of clinical trial research is to generate reliable information that can resolve the current state of clinical equipoise while protecting the interests of study participants [17]. While many would not challenge the merits of randomisation as a tool for clinical trial research, it can be uncomfortable since randomisation (and other design features) alters the way participants are treated [19, 20]. Instead of recommendations from a treating clinician with an ethical duty to provide the best possible care, random chance determines what a participant receives even when the assigned treatment may conflict with the individual recommendation [21]. Even so, clinical equipoise guarantees that no participant in randomised clinical trials receives care that is known to be inferior to available alternatives [21].

Design Type

Parallel Group and Crossover Designs

In clinical trials with parallel group design, subjects are randomised to a study arm, and they remain on the assigned arm for the duration of the study. In a two-arm parallel trial, patients would be allocated to either intervention A or B and remain on the assigned study arm for the duration of the study. In a crossover design, on the other hand, subjects are randomised to a sequence of treatments in which they cross over from one treatment to another during the trial. In a two-arm crossover trial, patients would be allocated to a sequence of AB or BA. In the crossover between the initially administered intervention to the other intervention, there is a washout period intended to eliminate the effects of the initial intervention.

Multi-Arm and Factorial Designs

Multi-arm designs refer to a type of trial design that has more than two arms in the clinical trial. In contrast to two-arm designs, where a single experimental intervention arm is usually compared against a control group that consists of active control or placebo, multi-arm designs involve multiple experimental interventions being compared to a shared control group or against each other directly in a head-to-head comparison. Conducting a single multi-arm clinical trial can be faster and cheaper than conducting a series of two-arm clinical trials, but multi-arm designs are not as commonly used as two-arm designs [22].

Factorial designs refer to a type of trial design that simultaneously evaluates the effect of two or more interventions using various combinations of interventions [23]. For instance, in a 2×2 factorial trial, participants are randomised to one of the four combinations of two interventions (A and B). Here, the combination of these intervention strategies (A alone; B alone; and A+B combined) can be compared against a control arm that does not receive either intervention A or B (no A nor B). Factorial designs can be appealing since two or more interventions can be assessed in the same population simultaneously [24]. Assuming that there is no interaction between the interventions, factorial designs can be an efficient way to test multiple interventions. Factorial designs may also allow for testing of the treatment interactions, but this typically requires a considerably larger sample size [24].

Fixed Sample Trial Design

In fixed sample trial designs, also commonly referred as conventional or traditional designs, the trial data are only analysed once, when the trials are finished after a priori determined sample size has been reached [25–27]. Clinical trials with fixed sample trial designs are designed with a fixed maximum sample size, a fixed number of interventions, and a defined end to the trial. This approach is relatively straightforward, since it involves three general steps of trial design, trial conduct as prescribed by the design outlined the trial protocol, and final analysis according to the pre-specified analysis plan once the target sample size is reached [1]. Fixed trial designs do not plan for modifications to major design components (e.g., sample size, allocation ratio) that may become desirable or necessary during the course of the trial [25–27].

Adaptive Trial Design

'Adaptive trial design' is a clinical trial design umbrella term that offers pre-specified opportunities to modify aspects of an ongoing trial based on accumulating trial data [28, 29]. In adaptive clinical trials, one or more 'interim analyses' are used to evaluate the trial data from an ongoing trial, and based on the results of the interim analysis, trial design features such as allocation ratio, sample size, and eligibility can be modified. Adaptive trial designs are a data-driven approach to clinical trial evaluation that allows for the trial to learn before a priori targeted sample size or number of events has been reached. The design of adaptive clinical trials would include pre-specification of number and frequency of interim analyses and statistical thresholds and rules for adaptation (decision rules). We will discuss the concept of adaptive trial designs and different types of adaptive trial design in the upcoming chapters.

Master Protocols

The term 'master protocols' (also sometimes referred to as core protocols) generally refers to an overarching protocol designed to evaluate multiple interventional hypotheses. There is usually a set of protocol documents with standardised operating procedures outlined. The framework of a master protocol aims to improve data collection through harmonisation of trial procedures with common standardised operating procedures that are then implemented across multiple different institutions with centralised governance structure. While this terminology refers to a set of protocol documents, people usually use this terminology to describe three types of clinical trial designs: 'platform trials', 'basket trials', and 'umbrella trials'. In this book, we will refer to master protocols as protocol documents and use the framework of master protocols as a way of harmonising clinical trial research.

Platform Trials, Basket Trials, and Umbrella Trials

Platform trials are a type of randomised clinical trial design in which multiple interventions can be evaluated simultaneously against a common control group with flexibilities of allowing new interventions to be added and the control group to be updated throughout the trial [30]. Platform trials use a master protocol to streamline and improve the quality of many of the trial processes and logistics [31]. These trials typically compare multiple interventions against a common control group using prespecified interim analysis plans for statistical efficiencies.

Basket trials refer to clinical trials in which a targeted therapy is evaluated for multiple diseases with a common risk factor, such as a molecular alteration, or risk factors that may help predict whether patients will respond to the given therapy (target of treatable trait) [31]. Umbrella trials refer to clinical trials that evaluate multiple targeted therapies in a single disease that is stratified into multiple sub-studies based on different molecular or other predictive risk factors [31]. Both basket and umbrella trials can be platform trials in nature if they are designed to have a common control group and enable the addition of new interventions during the trial. A key element of these trials is use of a master protocol.

Trial Planning

Trial Protocol

Clinical trials are based on a protocol document that details the study rationale, methods, organisation, ethical consideration, and other research plans. Trial protocols are used to document plans for study conduct from participant recruitment, randomisation plan, data analysis, to results dissemination, and other research plans. High-quality trial protocols can facilitate proper preparation, conduct, reporting, and external review of clinical trials [32]. The SPIRIT (Standard Protocol Items: Recommendations for Interventional Trials) Statement outlines key trial protocol elements [32]; there is also a website of resources (www .spirit-statement.org) that can help with drafting of trial protocols.

Estimands

The International Council for Harmonisation of Technical Requirements for Pharmaceuticals for Human Use (ICH) is a global organisation that brings together regulatory authorities and the pharmaceutical industry to ensure development and registration of high-quality medicines. ICH issues numerous guidance documents used internationally in the design and conduct of clinical trials. A key guideline relating to design and analysis of clinical trials is ICH *E9 Statistical Principals for Clinical Trials*. In November 2019, ICH has issued the final version of an addendum (R1) to ICH E9, ICH E9(R1), which introduced the concept of the estimand framework to precisely describe the treatment effect of interest in clinical trials [33].

An estimand refers to a target estimation to address the scientific question of interest posed by the trial objective (i.e., what is to be estimated) [33]. As objective setting is a necessary early step in the development of a clinical trial, the choice of objectives directly lead to the estimands [34]. The choice and specification of estimands should be defined early on during the planning stage [34]. Once there are well-defined estimands, clear trial objectives can be translated into key scientific questions, and a suitable method of estimation ('estimator') and numerical results ('estimate') can be selected [33].

An estimand has five attributes: (1) the population targeted by the scientific question; (2) treatment strategy, (3) endpoint (variable) to be measured for each patient, (4) strategies of handling intercurrent events, and (5) population-level summary measure [33]. The term 'outcome' refers to the measured variable (e.g., mortality), whereas an 'endpoint' refers to an analysed parameter of a given outcome (e.g., survival at 28 days since randomisation). 'Intercurrent events' refer to events occurring post-randomisation that preclude or affect the interpretation or the existence of measurement associated with the clinical question of interest [33]. Examples of intercurrent events include premature discontinuation of the assigned treatment, initiation of rescue therapy, or switch to an alternate therapy [33, 35].

There are different strategies for handling intercurrent events. Prior to the ICH E9(R1) guideline, intention-to-treat (ITT) and per-protocol (PP) principles were the most common approach to statistical analyses. In an ITT analysis, all patients are analysed in accordance to the group to which they were randomly assigned, regardless of whether they received the assigned therapy [36]. ITT analyses can be viewed as 'as-randomised' analyses. In a PP analysis, only data from participants who follow the protocol are used, and data from patients who did not adhere to the protocol are excluded [36]. PP analyses can be subject to bias, since lack of adherence is often non-random, and between patients who adhere to the protocol versus those who do not may differ in important prognostic characteristics that influence their outcomes [37].

The ICH E9(R1) guideline discusses five common strategies for handling intercurrent events: (1) 'treatment policy strategy', (2) 'composite strategy', (3) 'hypothetical strategy', (4) 'while on treatment strategy', and (5) 'principal stratum strategy' [33]. In the *treatment policy strategy*, the occurrence of the intercurrent is considered irrelevant, and the data collected for the variable of interest are used regardless of whether any intercurrent events occur or not [33]. The treatment policy strategy is closely related to the ITT principle [33]. In the *composite strategy*, the intercurrent event is integrated as a component of the variable [33]. For instance, the variable might be defined as a composite outcome consisting of no rescue therapy use and a favourable clinical outcome, so a patient is considered a non-responder if they need to use rescue medication and/or if they have a non-favourable outcome [33].

In the *hypothetical strategy*, a hypothetical scenario is envisaged in which the intercurrent event does not occur. Under the hypothetical strategy, the observed outcome of patients without intercurrent events corresponds to the outcome of interest, but the outcome of patients who experience intercurrent events, since the hypothetical scenario cannot be observed, is considered as missing and imputed [36]. In the *while on treatment strategy*, response to treatment prior to the occurrence of the intercurrent event is of interest [33]. If a variable is measured repeatedly, its value up to the time of the intercurrent event may be included in the analysis to account for the intercurrent event. In the *principal stratum strategy*, subpopulations of interest are defined according to the potential occurrence of an intercurrent event on one or all treatments [39]. The subpopulations could be based on who would tolerate treatment if assigned to the treatment. Among studies where the estimand framework is explicitly adopted, the treatment policy strategy is the most common estimand, and there are currently only a few studies using the other strategies.

For the population-level summary measure, it is important to cover both within study-arm and (if applicable) between study-arm summaries [34]. An example of within study-arm summary measures included a proportion of patients alive at 28 days, and corresponding examples of between study-arm summaries could include odds ratio, risk ratio, or absolute risk difference. The population-level summary measure is specific to the choice in endpoint. If time-to-event endpoint for an outcome of mortality is used, overall survival would be the within study-arm summary measure and the hazard ratio (HR) is the standard summary measure for between study-arm summary measure.

Sample Size and Statistical Power Determination

Determination of sample size and statistical power is a fundamental step for clinical trial design. Clinical trials should be planned with sufficiently large sample size that allows for high statistical power to detect clinically important treatment effects. Before a discussion on statistical power and sample size, it should be emphasised that a sample size calculation only provides an estimate of the size of the trial. The sample size calculations require specification of the desired statistical power, level of significance (alpha), the variability of the endpoint being studied, the size of treatment effects of interest, and the anticipated loss to follow-up. Sample size calculations are most often a guesstimate because there is often a large uncertainty in the parameters required in the sample size calculations.

Statistical power informally refers to the probability of detecting an effect if there is a true effect. Statistical power is the complement of a type II error (false negative error rate) that refers to an error of failing to reject the null hypothesis when it should be (false negative finding): *Power = 1 − type II error rate*. A null hypothesis is a type of conjecture used in hypothesis testing that proposes there is no difference between two or more groups.

All else being equal, sample size requirements will increase with power. The level of significance is usually referred to as type I error rate (false positive error rate) that researchers are willing to accept. Type I error refers to the error of rejecting the null hypothesis when it is true. Even though it is arbitrary, the convention in clinical trial research is to use 80% statistical power and an alpha of 5%. Eighty per cent power means that if everything in the trial goes as planned and given that there is a true treatment effect, there is an 80% chance of observing a statistically significant result and a 20% chance of not being able to reject the null hypothesis. An alpha of 5% implies that one is willing to accept a 5% chance of a type I error rate in their clinical trial, should the null hypothesis be true. When planning an RCT with a dichotomous endpoint, the sample size calculation requires pre-specification of type I error rate and statistical power, control event rates, desired or expected treatment effects, and the rate of attrition.

Simulation

Simulation in statistics generally refers to repeated analyses of randomly generated datasets with known properties [40]. Datasets are repeatedly drawn using computer software under assumptions made on the data-generating mechanism and design specifications [40]. In the context of trials planning, clinical trial simulations refer to a large number of computer-generated runs performed under various assumptions to evaluate the trial's operating characteristics such as type I error rate, power, expected sample size, and duration [41]. Clinical trial simulations are useful for trial planning since they allow evaluation of a multitude of potential scenarios that may occur during the trial. With many unknowns and assumptions that need to be made at the trial planning stage, clinical trial simulations can help to avoid trial design decisions that trial investigators would regret later after the trial shows negative findings (areas of 'anticipated regret') [42]. In our opinion, clinical trial simulations are useful for all trial designs. Even though techniques for estimating sample sizes for conventional fixed sample trials are well established, the use of clinical trial simulations allows for considerations of multiple design options as candidate designs in the planning stage. Clinical trial simulations could be used to compare a fixed trial design option to different adaptive trial designs.

Clinical trial simulations are more commonly used in adaptive trial designs because decision-making processes are often complex and statistical properties are difficult to evaluate without simulations [43]. Closed form expressions, such as mathematical equations for sample size calculations, cannot be derived for many of adaptive trial designs, so simulations are usually required. For planning of adaptive trial designs, clinical trial simulations are needed to investigate different possible scenarios and help predict the likelihood of potential adaptations and their consequences on performance characteristics of the design [43]. Clinical trial simulation helps to estimate the performance of different study modifications and decision rules, using metrics such as expected reduction in required sample size and time to completion, number of treatment failures avoided, treatment effect estimate biases, risk of drop-outs or other noncompliance, and robustness of planned statistical analysis. Clinical trial simulations are ideal to evaluate the trade-offs between the potential benefits and risks between different adaptations that are being considered by the investigators. We will revisit the concept of simulations and their utility in Chapter 5.

Statistical Framework

Frequentist versus Bayesian Statistics

There are two competing statistical philosophies: the frequentist and Bayesian statistics. Frequentist methods regard population values, such as population means and proportions, as a fixed but unknown quantity, without a probability distribution. Frequentists then perform significance tests of hypotheses (usually the null hypothesis) concerning it or calculates confidence intervals for this quantity [44]. In a Bayesian framework, on the other hand, these population values are viewed as random and therefore Bayesians assign probability distributions to them [44, 45]. For example, frequentists would say a response rate under a given treatment is 30%, and Bayesians would say the treatment response is most likely 30% but could be anywhere between 15% and 45%.

Since frequentist statistics are most used in clinical trial research and other types of research, most readers may likely be familiar with the frequentist approach and concepts such as p-values and confidence intervals. The p-value refers to the probability under a specified statistical analysis that a statistical summary of the data (e.g., sample mean difference between two compared groups) would be at least as extreme as its observed value [46]. The p-value is the probability that the chosen test statistic would have been as extreme as observed if all model assumptions were correct including the hypothesis being tested [47]. The null hypothesis that postulates the absence of treatment effect is the most often targeted hypothesis. A low p-value in this context can be used as evidence against the null hypothesis, such that when the p-value is below 0.05 (or other pre-specified 'significance' threshold), we can use it to reject the null hypothesis. While p-values can be a useful statistical measure, it is often misinterpreted [47]. Therefore, p-values *do not* indicate the probability that the data were produced by random chance alone nor do they measure the probability that the null hypothesis is true. A p-value of 0.01 does not indicate that there is only a 1% chance of the null hypothesis of being true nor does it indicate that there is a 99% chance of the alternative hypothesis that postulates that there is a treatment effect of being true.

It has been discussed that shifting from p-values to confidence intervals will lead to fewer statistical misinterpretations. However, similar to p-values, the concept of confidence intervals is prone to misinterpretation [47]. Confidence interval estimate is a range of likely values for the population parameter. A 95% confidence interval tells us that if you were to (hypothetically) repeat the experiment infinite times, 95% of the intervals constructed would contain the true value of the population (if the model assumptions are correct). If we were to repeat the study 100 times and compute a 95% confidence interval in each study, then approximately 95 of the 100 confidence intervals will contain the true population parameter that we are trying to estimate. From a specific 95% confidence interval presented by a study, we cannot conclude that there is 95% probability that the treatment effect is between the upper and lower bounds of the confidence interval estimate [47]. In terms of frequentist statistics, the confidence interval either contains the population mean or it does not. The 95% confidence interval is a confidence that in the long run, 95% of the confidence intervals generated will include the population mean.

Bayesian statistics can estimate the (posterior) probability distributions of unknown parameters (e.g., treatment effects) using Bayes theorem. Here, the likelihood function that is based on the observed data can be combined with a prior probability distribution that represents our beliefs on plausible range of parameter values to estimate the posterior probability distributions that offer much more intuitive summaries. Instead of using p-values that indicate the compatibility between the observed data and the null hypothesis (and other aspects of the statistical model), using Bayesian statistics can estimate the posterior probability of an experiment intervention being superior to a control arm that is of direct interest to many research questions being evaluated in clinical trials [45, 48]. Instead of using confidence intervals that speak about the long-run confidence about hypothetical experiments, we can derive credible intervals that offer much more straight-forward interpretations. The 95% credible interval reflects the 95% probability that the unknown parameter is within an estimated interval. When we estimate 95% credible interval of clinical trial research, we can conclude that there is 95% probability that the estimated treatment effect is between the range indicated by the estimated interval.

Book Overview

An overview of our upcoming discussion of adaptive trial designs and master protocols in the book can be seen in Figure 1.1. While our discussion will primarily be based on randomised clinical trials, there are non-randomised trials that often use adaptive trial designs as well. There are important differences between adaptive trial and fixed sample trial designs, which will be discussed in upcoming chapters. Platform, basket, and umbrella trials that use a master protocol framework can be conducted with or without adaptive trial designs. It is a misconception that these trials will always be conducted with adaptive trial

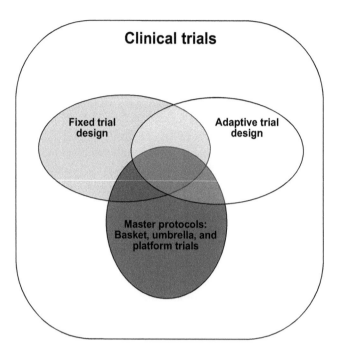

Figure 1.1 Overview of relationship between fixed trial designs, adaptive trial designs, and master protocols.

In this figure, an overlapping relationship between the three topics of this book in fixed trial design, adaptive trial design, and master protocols is provided.

designs. Figure 1.1 will become clearer for the reader as we review the concept of adaptive trial designs and master protocols in a detailed manner.

Conclusion

In this chapter, we have introduced the basic concepts of clinical research. We have distinguished clinical trials from observational studies and introduced the concepts of different clinical trial phases, value of randomisation and different randomisation techniques, design type, and a general overview of trial planning. The terminologies of adaptive trial designs and master protocols have been introduced as well as the concepts of frequentist and Bayesian statistics that are important for readers to understand in reading later chapters.

References

1. Friedman LM, Furberg C, DeMets DL, Reboussin D, Granger CB. *Fundamentals of Clinical Trials*: Springer; 2015.

2. Yuan J, Pang H, Tong T, et al. Seamless phase IIa/IIb and enhanced dose-finding adaptive design. *J Biopharm Stat*. 2016;**26**(5):912–23.

3. Malay S, Chung KC. The choice of controls for providing validity and evidence in clinical research. *Plast Reconstr Surg*. 2012;**130**(4):959–65.

4. Viele K, Berry S, Neuenschwander B, et al. Use of historical control data for assessing treatment effects in clinical trials. *Pharm Stat*. 2014;**13**(1):41–54.

5. Lachin JM. Statistical properties of randomization in clinical trials. *Control Clin Trials*. 1988;**9**(4):289–311.

6. Lachin JM, Matts JP, Wei LJ. Randomization in clinical trials: conclusions and recommendations. *Control Clin Trials*. 1988;**9**(4):365–74.

7. Cartwright N. What are randomised controlled trials good for? *Philos Stud*. 2010;**147**(1):59.

8. Senn S. Seven myths of randomisation in clinical trials. *Stat Med*. 2013;**32** (9):1439–50.

9. Deaton A, Cartwright N. Understanding and misunderstanding randomized controlled trials. *Soc Sci Med*. 2018;**210**:2–21.

10. Roberts C, Torgerson DJ. Understanding controlled trials: baseline imbalance in randomised controlled trials. *BMJ*. 1999;**319**(7203):185.

11. Broglio K. Randomization in clinical trials: permuted blocks and stratification. *JAMA*. 2018;**319**(21):2223–4.

12. McPherson GC, Campbell MK, Elbourne DR. Use of randomisation in clinical trials: a survey of UK practice. *Trials*. 2012;**13**(1):1–7.

13. Matts JP, Lachin JM. Properties of permuted-block randomization in clinical trials. *Control Clin Trials*. 1988;**9** (4):327–44.

14. Kang M, Ragan BG, Park JH. Issues in outcomes research: an overview of randomization techniques for clinical trials. *J Athl Train*. 2008;**43**(2):215–21.

15. Therneau TM. How many stratification factors are 'too many' to use in a randomization plan? *Control Clin trials*. 1993;**14**(2):98–108.

16. Kahan, BC, Morris, TP. Improper analysis of trials randomised using stratified blocks or minimisation. *Stat Med*. 2012;**31** (4):328–340.

17. Freedman B. Equipoise and the ethics of clinical research. *N Engl J Med*. 1987;**317** (3):141–5.

18. Cook C, Sheets C. Clinical equipoise and personal equipoise: two necessary ingredients for reducing bias in manual therapy trials. *J Man Manip Ther*. 2011;**19** (1):55–7.

19. Jepson M, Elliott D, Conefrey C, et al. An observational study showed that explaining randomization using gambling-related metaphors and computer-agency descriptions impeded randomized clinical trial recruitment. *J Clin Epidemiol*. 2018;**99**:75–83.

20. Angus DC. Optimizing the trade-off between learning and doing in a pandemic. *JAMA*. 2020;**323**(19):1895–6.

21. London AJ. Equipoise in research: integrating ethics and science in human research. *JAMA*. 2017;**317**(5):525–6.

22. Parmar MK, Carpenter J, Sydes MR. More multiarm randomised trials of superiority are needed. *Lancet*. 2014;**384**(9940):283–4.

23. Box GE, Hunter J, Hunter W. *Statistics for Experimenters. Design, Innovation and Discovery*, 2nd ed. John Wiley; 2005.

24. Montgomery AA, Peters TJ, Little P. Design, analysis and presentation of factorial randomised controlled trials. *BMC Med Res Methodol*. 2003;3:26.

25. Ondra T, Dmitrienko A, Friede T, et al. Methods for identification and confirmation of targeted subgroups in clinical trials: a systematic review. *J Biopharm Stat*. 2016;**26**(1):99–119.

26. Thorlund K, Haggstrom J, Park JJ, Mills EJ. Key design considerations for adaptive clinical trials: a primer for clinicians. *BMJ*. 2018;**360**:k698.

27. Park JJ, Thorlund K, Mills EJ. Critical concepts in adaptive clinical trials. *Clin Epidemiol*. 2018;**10**:343–51.

28. Dimairo M, Pallmann P, Wason J et al. The Adaptive designs CONSORT Extension (ACE) statement: a checklist with explanation and elaboration guideline for reporting randomised trials that use an adaptive design. *BMJ*. 2020;**369**:m115.

29. Dimairo M, Pallmann P, Wason J, et al. The Adaptive designs CONSORT extension (ACE) statement: a checklist with explanation and elaboration guideline for reporting randomised trials that use an adaptive design. *Trials*. 2020;**21**(1):528.

30. Adaptive Platform Trials Coalition. Adaptive platform trials: definition, design,

conduct and reporting considerations. *Nat Rev Drug Discov* 2019;**18**(10):797–807.

31. Woodcock J, LaVange LM. Master protocols to study multiple therapies, multiple diseases, or both. *N Engl J Med.* 2017;**377**(1):62–70.

32. Chan AW, Tetzlaff JM, Gotzsche PC, et al. SPIRIT 2013 explanation and elaboration: guidance for protocols of clinical trials. *BMJ.* 2013;346:e7586.

33. International Council for Harmonisation of Technical Requirements for Pharmaceuticals for Human Use. *Addendum on Estimands and Sensitivity Analysis in Clinical Trials to the Guideline on Statistical Principles for Clinical Trials E9(R1)*; 2019. https://database.ich.org/sites/default/files/E9-R1_Step4_Guideline_2019_1203.pdf

34. Bell J, Hamilton A, Sailer O, Voss F. The detailed clinical objectives approach to designing clinical trials and choosing estimands. *Pharm Stat.* 2021;**20**(6):1112–24.

35. Ratitch B, Goel N, Mallinckrodt C, et al. Defining efficacy estimands in clinical trials: examples illustrating ICH E9(R1) guidelines. *Ther Innov Regul Sci.* 2020;**54**(2):370–84.

36. Smith VA, Coffman CJ, Hudgens MG. Interpreting the results of intention-to-treat, per-protocol, and as-treated analyses of clinical trials. *JAMA.* 2021;**326**(5):433–4.

37. Sussman JB, Hayward RA. An IV for the RCT: using instrumental variables to adjust for treatment contamination in randomised controlled trials. *BMJ (Clinical Res Ed).* 2010;**340**:c2073.

38. Parra CO, Daniel RM, Bartlett JW. Hypothetical estimands in clinical trials: a unification of causal inference and missing data methods. *arXiv preprint arXiv*:210704392. 2021.

39. Bornkamp B, Rufibach K, Lin J, et al. Principal stratum strategy: potential role in drug development. *Pharm Stat.* 2021;**20**(4):737–51.

40. Burton A, Altman DG, Royston P, Holder RL. The design of simulation studies in medical statistics. *Stat Med.* 2006;**25**(24):4279–92.

41. Holford N, Ma SC, Ploeger BA. Clinical trial simulation: a review. *Clin Pharm Therap.* 2010;**88**(2):166–82.

42. U.S. Food and Drug Administration. *Adaptive Designs for Medical Device Clinical Studies Guidance for Industry and Food and Drug Administration Staff.* United States Department of Health and Human Services; 2016.

43. Hummel J, Wang S, Kirkpatrick J. Using simulation to optimize adaptive trial designs: applications in learning and confirmatory phase trials. *Clin Investig.* 2015;**5**(4):401–13.

44. Bland JM, Altman DG. Bayesians and frequentists. *BMJ.* 1998;**317**(7166):1151–60.

45. Berry DA. Bayesian clinical trials. *Nat Rev Drug Discov.* 2006;**5**(1):27–36.

46. Wasserstein RL, Lazar NA. *The ASA Statement on p-Values: Context, Process, and Purpose.* Taylor & Francis; 2016. pp. 129–33.

47. Greenland S, Senn SJ, Rothman KJ, et al. Statistical tests, P values, confidence intervals, and power: a guide to misinterpretations. *Eur J Epidemiol.* 2016;**31**(4):337–50.

48. Gill CJ, Sabin L, Schmid CH. Why clinicians are natural Bayesians. *BMJ.* 2005;**330**(7499):1080–3.

Chapter 2

History of Clinical Trial Research

Jay J. H. Park, J. Kyle Wathen, and Edward J. Mills

Key Points of This Chapter

In this chapter, we succinctly discuss the history of clinical trials, adaptive trial designs, and master protocols. The key points of this chapter are:

- The history of clinical trials follows a long journey. The discipline of randomised clinical trials was born out of economic hardship.
- No experiments can be perfect. Nuanced discussions are required to consider the trade-offs between scientific, economic, and other practical constraints in the design stage. Critical evaluation of evidence generated from each clinical trial requires nuanced appraisal.

Introduction

Over the years, the discipline of clinical trials has made important methodological advances in adaptive trial designs and master protocols, the two main topics of this book. Before we investigate the topics of adaptive trial designs and master protocols in greater detail in later chapters, in this chapter, we look at the history and landmark clinical trials that have shaped the fundamental design and implementation of clinical trial research. The current practices of medicine and public health are inherently connected to the discipline of clinical trials, and randomised clinical trials are established as the standard mechanism for generating evidence on the effectiveness of therapeutic interventions in medical research. The history of clinical trials tells us that this was not always the case.

History of Clinical Trials

The 1948 Streptomycin Trial for Tuberculosis

The birth of randomised clinical trials dates back to 1948 when the United Kingdom (UK) Medical Research Council (MRC) randomised clinical trial of streptomycin for pulmonary tuberculosis was published [1]. Credit for randomised clinical trials is usually given to Sir Austin Bradford Hill, a professor of Medical Statistics who designed and helped conduct this trial. This landmark trial has paved the way for randomised clinical trials now being widely accepted as the gold standard for clinical research [2]. But it was different back in the 1940s. At least 10 years earlier, Hill had been advocating for strictly controlled experiments with groups being chosen at random [3–5]. Hill deliberately left out the word 'randomisation' in the first edition of his handbook *Principle of Medical Statistics* published in the *Lancet* in 1937 when he was trying to persuade doctors to adopt controlled clinical trials [3, 4]. Randomisation was then a foreign statistical concept to the medical community [3].

The MRC streptomycin trial occurred shortly after World War II. This was a time of immense resource limitations and widespread illnesses and injuries. Tuberculosis was one of the leading causes of mortality among young adults in Europe and North America [6]. In 1943, streptomycin was discovered by Albert Schatz and Selman Waksman and proved to be effective against a bacterium (*Mycobacterium tuberculosis*) that causes tuberculosis in the test tube and in guinea pigs [7]. Since the war had effectively stripped the UK of financial resources, the local government could afford to purchase streptomycin for only a limited number of patients (55 to be exact) [3, 6]. According to Hill, this shortage due to economic hardship was the dominant reason that this first randomised clinical trial was possible [3]. The MRC could justify that the limited drug supply could be fairly allocated if it was used in a rigorously planned randomised clinical trial with concurrent control [3].

While Hill has passed away in 1991, the legacy of MRC streptomycin trial still lives on. This trial arguably marks the start of new era with randomised clinical trials acting as the centrepiece of medicine. It is easy to forget how the concept so central to current practice of medicine in randomisation could have been rejected.

The History of Adaptive Trial Designs

The ECMO Trials

The first influential adaptive clinical trial we can think of can be tracked back to 1985 when Robert H. Bartlett and colleagues published their trial that tested the effectiveness of extracorporeal membrane oxygenation (ECMO) procedure as a treatment with newborns with respiratory failure [8]. ECMO is a heart-lung bypass procedure intended for life-threatening cardiac or pulmonary failures. Conducting a randomised clinical trial on a vulnerable population such those newborns who require ECMO has its challenges. It is not easy to communicate to the family, even at random, why their newborn has been assigned to a conventional treatment and not the experimental treatment that is being tested. Randomisation can also be profoundly uncomfortable for clinicians prescribing unproven therapy to vulnerable populations whom they have sworn to treat to the best of their ability [9].

When Bartlett and colleagues conducted their randomised clinical trial with the play-the-winner allocation method on ECMO, they used this design to balance the challenges of withholding a potentially lifesaving treatment without disrupting the experimental nature of their randomised clinical trial [8]. The play-the-winner method was proposed by Zelen [10] in 1969 and Wei and Durham [11] in 1978, but had never before been used in a clinical study. Under the play-the-winner method, the first patient has an equal chance of being randomised to either treatment A or B. If treatment A is selected and is successful, the next patient is more likely randomised to that treatment, whereas if treatment A is unsuccessful, the next patient is more likely randomised to the other treatment. The allocation was done using sealed envelopes; the statistician responsible for adapting the allocation ratio did not know which assignment (A or B) corresponded to ECMO. In this trial, the first neonate who ended up

Table 2.1 Findings from O'Rourke et al., 1989 [12]

Mortality	ECMO arm	Control arm
Stage 1	0/9 (0.0%)	4/10 (40.0%)
Stage 2	1/20 (5.0%)	–
Overall mortality rate	1/29 (3.4%)	4/10 (40.0%)

Data are n/N (%).

receiving the standard-of-care died. Then the second neonate randomised to ECMO survived along with the subsequent 10 neonates who were assigned to ECMO [8].

Following the Bartlett et al. study, Pearl O'Rourke and colleagues [12] conducted another adaptive clinical trial with the two-stage approach. Instead of using play-the-winner or other forms of response adaptive randomisation, O'Rourke et al. conducted a trial with two phases. In the first stage, neonates were randomly assigned to ECMO or standard-of-care (control) at an equal allocation ratio until there were four deaths observed in either group; at the second stage of this trial, all patients would be assigned to the more successful treatment until either four deaths were observed in that group or until statistical significance was achieved [12]. In the first stage, 9 neonates who were randomly assigned to the ECMO arm all survived, whereas out of the 10 neonates assigned to the control, 4 died (Table 2.1). As planned, the trial transitioned into the second stage where 1 out of 20 more neonates treated ECMO arm ended up dying.

These ECMO trials have been criticised at both ends of the spectrum. They were criticised because some believed no neonates with these critical conditions should have received the standard therapy, and others criticised these trials for using an 'adaptive design' that could have biased the results [13]. The UK Collaborative ECMO Trial Group was one of these groups that criticised the two adaptive trials by Bartlett's play-the-winner design and O'Rourke's two-stage design for becoming more lenient towards ECMO over time and including a limited number of neonates in the control group [13]. In response, the UK Collaborative ECMO Trial Group conducted a randomised clinical trial using equal allocation between ECMO and the control with the maximum sample size of 300 neonates. The trial recruitment started in January 1993, and in November 1995, the Data and Safety Monitoring Board (DSMB) made a recommendation to the Trial Steering Committee that the trial had to stop when 180 neonates (~62% planned sample size) had been observed for an outcome [13]. The Trial Steering Committee met 10 days later and decided that the trial provided a clear answer and could be stopped early for superiority of ECMO over the control arm (Table 2.2).

The UK Collaborative ECMO Trial was made possible due to large, collaborative participation from hundreds of clinicians and parents and affected neonates with life-threatening conditions. Perhaps after reading the results from their convincing trial results, it is easy to be judgemental and say this large trial should never have been conducted. No clinical trial is perfect after all, but perhaps there is a need to better optimise the trade-off between the experimental nature of clinical trials and clinical practice [9].

Table 2.2 Findings from the UK Collaborative ECMO Trial [13]

Outcome	ECMO arm	Control arm
Mortality	33/93 (35%)	54/92 (59%)
Risk ratio (95% CI)	0.60 (0.44, 0.84)	1.00 (reference group)

Data are n/N (%) and risk ratio for the mortality outcome. The final published data included data from 185 neonates instead of 180 neonates when the interim report was provided to the DSMB. CI, confidence interval.

Development of Master Protocols

Compared to the history of randomised clinical trials and adaptive trial designs, the concept of master protocols is arguably in its infancy. The concept and framework of 'master protocols' have initially been motivated and developed from the field of oncology. The advancements in genomics, particularly in tumour sequencing, have improved our ability to differentiate cancers by their genetic mutations and fuelled the efforts towards 'precision oncology', where therapies are selected to specifically target cancers based on their genetic mutations [14, 15]. Over the past decade, this has not only helped motivate the work towards precision oncology but also motivated the development of master protocols, since it is unrealistic to investigate the broad spectrum of genetic sub-populations by conventional trial designs. Thus, the master protocol framework has been proposed to provide a means of comprehensively and adaptively evaluating treatments from the field of precision oncology [16, 17].

The first review article describing the concept of master protocols was written by Redman and Allegra in 2015 [16]. They described the need to test multiple new targeted agents and need to develop novel therapeutic platforms where multiple targeted therapies can be tested in lung cancer patients. Master protocols had received support from the U.S. Food and Drug Administration (FDA) early on. In 2018, the FDA released its draft guidance document outlining recommendations for master protocols, and basket, umbrella, and platform trials [18]. Prior to this, Janet Woodcock and Lisa LaVange, who were at the time acting as the directors of the FDA's Center for Drug Evaluation and Research (CDER), published their 2017 editorial, which many consider the hallmark paper of master protocol, titled 'Master Protocols to Study Multiple Therapies, Multiple Diseases, or Both' in the *New England Journal of Medicine* [19].

The framework of master protocols can be tailored and adapted to suit the research objectives' multiple clinical indications. However, as the development of master protocols originated from the field of oncology, the initial application was largely limited to other areas of research [20]. Since basket and umbrella trials typically involve evaluation of targeted therapies that require strong genomic biomarker characterisation, they are still very much limited to oncology. Platform trials that allow interventions to enter and leave the trial infrastructure at different times are increasingly being used outside of oncology [21].

The momentum and enthusiasm towards platform trials came largely after the novel coronavirus disease 2019 (COVID-19) pandemic [22]. In hopes of returning to normalcy, the world has looked to the scientific community for the rapid discovery of treatment and preventive measures against COVID-19. For the pandemic, clinical trials needed to be nimble and dynamic to adapt to new internal and external scientific discoveries that reflected in rapidly changing standard-of-care and practice [23]. The medical community saw conclusive evidence from many COVID-19 platform trials, while the majority of conventional (non-platform) trials were largely disappointing [22, 24]. As we saw with the COVID-19 pandemic, large platform trials are the ideal choice for clinical trial research aiming to determine the most effective therapy for an indication.

Conclusion

Since the start of randomised clinical trials, important methodological advancements, notably in adaptive trial designs and master protocols, have been made to offset limitations that conventional trial designs can pose [20, 25–27]. Similar to how the concept of randomisation was once, the concepts of adaptive trial designs and master protocols remain as foreign concepts to many members of the medical community. Based on our experience working in the field of clinical trial research, one dominant reason for the expressed opposition to these newer approaches could be a lack of understanding. This failure of understanding is not due to a paucity of information. There is a vast literature about adaptive trial designs and, recently, master protocols describing their purpose, methods, and strengths and limitations. As much of that literature has been written using technical jargon, it is not surprising that these concepts are often misinterpreted.

Now that we have finished our brief review of history, we can proceed to the next chapters for more in-depth and focused discussion of adaptive trial designs and master protocols.

References

1. Bothwell LE, Podolsky SH. The emergence of the randomized, controlled trial. *N Engl J Med.* 2016;**375**(6):501–4.

2. Jones DS, Podolsky SH. The history and fate of the gold standard. *Lancet.* 2015;**385** (9977):1502–3.

3. Hill AB. Suspended judgment. Memories of the British Streptomycin Trial in Tuberculosis. The first randomized clinical trial. *Control Clin Trials.* 1990;**11**(2):77–9.

4. Hill AB. *Principles of Medical Statistics.* 1st ed. *Lancet.* 1937.

5. Hill AB. I. – The aim of the statistical method. *Lancet.* 1937;**229**(5914):41–3.

6. Crofton J. The MRC randomized trial of streptomycin and its legacy: a view from the clinical front line. *J R Soc Med.* 2006;**99** (10):531–4.

7. Schatz A, Waksman SA. Effect of streptomycin and other antibiotic substances upon *Mycobacterium tuberculosis* and related organisms. *Proc Soc Exp Biol Med.* 1944;**57**(2):244–8.

8. Bartlett RH, Roloff DW, Cornell RG, et al. Extracorporeal circulation in neonatal respiratory failure: a prospective randomized study. *Pediatrics.* 1985;**76** (4):479–87.

9. Angus DC. Optimizing the trade-off between learning and doing in a pandemic. *JAMA.* 2020;**323**(19):1895–6.

10. Zelen M. Play the winner rule and the controlled clinical trial. *J Am Stat Assoc.* 1969;**64**(325):131–46.

11. Wei L, Durham S. The randomized play-the-winner rule in medical trials. *J Am Stat Assoc.* 1978;**73**(364):840–3.

12. O'Rourke PP, Crone RK, Vacanti JP, et al. Extracorporeal membrane oxygenation and conventional medical therapy in neonates with persistent pulmonary hypertension of the newborn: a prospective

randomized study. *Pediatrics.* 1989;**84** (6):957–63.

13. UK Collaborative ECMO Trial Group. UK Collaborative Randomised Trial of Neonatal Extracorporeal Membrane Oxygenation. *Lancet.* 1996;**348** (9020):75–82.

14. Kumar-Sinha C, Chinnaiyan AM. Precision oncology in the age of integrative genomics. *Nat Biotechnol.* 2018;**36** (1):46–60.

15. Ke X, Shen L. Molecular targeted therapy of cancer: the progress and future prospect. *Front Lab Med.* 2017;**1**(2):69–75.

16. Redman MW, Allegra CJ. The master protocol concept. *Semin Oncol.* 2015;**42** (5):724–30.

17. Hirakawa A, Asano J, Sato H, Teramukai S. Master protocol trials in oncology: review and new trial designs. *Contemp Clin Trials Commun.* 2018;**12**:1–8.

18. U.S. Department of Health and Human Services, U.S. Food and Drug Administration. *Master Protocols: Efficient Clinical Trial Design Strategies to Expedite Development of Oncology Drugs and Biologics Guidance for Industry (Draft Guidance).* United States Department of Health and Human Services; 2018. www.fda.gov/downloads/Drugs/ GuidanceComplianceRegulatory Information/Guidances/UCM621817.pdf

19. Woodcock J, LaVange LM. Master protocols to study multiple therapies, multiple diseases, or both. *N Engl J Med.* 2017;**377**(1):62–70.

20. Park JJH, Siden E, Zoratti MJ, et al. Systematic review of basket trials, umbrella trials, and platform trials: a landscape analysis of master protocols. *Trials.* 2019;**20**(1):572.

21. Bogin V. Master protocols: new directions in drug discovery. *Contemp Clin Trials Commun.* 2020;**18**:100568.

22. Vanderbeek AM, Bliss JM, Yin Z, Yap C. Implementation of platform trials in the COVID-19 pandemic: a rapid review. *Contemp Clin Trials.* 2022;**112**:106625.

23. Park JJ, Mogg R, Smith GE, et al. How COVID-19 has fundamentally changed clinical research in global health. *Lancet Glob Health.* 2021;**9**(5):e711–e20.

24. Park JJH, Dron L, Mills EJ. Moving forward in clinical research with master protocols. *Contemp Clin Trials.* 2021;**106**:106438.

25. Armitage P. Sequential medical trials. *Biomedicine.* 1978;28 Spec No:40–1.

26. Bauer P, Bretz F, Dragalin V, Konig F, Wassmer G. Twenty-five years of confirmatory adaptive designs: opportunities and pitfalls. *Stat Med.* 2016;**35**(3):325–47.

27. Woodcock J, LaVange LM. Master protocols to study multiple therapies, multiple diseases, or both. *N Engl J Med.* 2017; **377**(1):62–70.

Characteristics and Principles of Adaptive Trial Designs

Jay J. H. Park, J. Kyle Wathen, and Edward J. Mills

Key Points of This Chapter

This chapter discusses the property and principles of adaptive trial designs. The key points of this chapter are:

- Adaptive trial designs refer to trial designs that offer pre-planned opportunities to modify design of an ongoing trial based on accumulating trial data.
- Decisions for potential adaptations are made during the trial based on interim data, but flexibilities in adaptive trial designs are established and outlined in the study documents before any patient is recruited.
- For statistical planning, a simulation-guided approach is often used to evaluate the statistical properties of the design. It is generally required to demonstrate control of false positive rates for the regulatory, ethics, and funding bodies.
- Measures to mitigate and plan for operational bias and complexity in adaptive trial designs are needed.

Introduction

Conventional clinical trials, also commonly referred to as fixed sample trial design, involve a single analysis being conducted when a priori sample size (or number of events) has been reached. At the design stage, these trials often involve sample size calculations in which the investigators must make assumptions about the population, interventions, outcomes, and other trial parameters based on information that is available at the planning stage. The success of clinical trials is often dependent on the accuracy of these parameters used to plan the design, but there are often uncertainties in these assumptions. Fixed sample size designs do not enable options for modifications, but they may become desirable after the trial starts.

As an alternative to conventional designs, adaptive trial designs can be used to manage uncertainties surrounding the 'informed guesses' that are required during the design stage. 'Adaptive trial design' is an overarching term for clinical trial designs that offer pre-planned opportunities to modify aspects of an ongoing trial based on accumulating trial data [1, 2]. Adaptive trial designs can be applied across all phases of clinical research (phase I to phase III) to make clinical trials more flexible and responsive to accumulating trial data. They are a data-driven approach to clinical trial research that allows for the trial to learn and modify aspects of its design based on the results of 'interim' trial data [3]. In this chapter, we discuss key concepts and terminologies of adaptive trial designs and the unifying characteristics and important principles related to their design and conduct.

Important Concepts and Terminologies of Adaptive Trial Designs

Glossary

- **Adaptive trial design** refers to clinical trial designs that offer pre-planned opportunities to modify aspects of an ongoing trial based on accumulating trial data
- **Blinded analysis** (synonym: non-comparative analysis) refers to an analysis that is done while maintaining blinding of the treatment allocation
- **Data safety monitoring board** (synonym: data monitoring committee) is an independent group of experts who monitor the progress of a clinical trial and review safety and effectiveness data while the trial is ongoing.
- **Fixed sample trial design** (synonym: conventional trial design) refers to clinical trial designs with a target sample size or number of events that are not subject to pre-specified adaptations.
- **Independent statistical analysis centre** (synonym: independent statisticians) refers to individuals responsible for the statistical analysis of trial data including interim analyses. The independent statistical analysis centre often prepares reports for an independent data safety monitoring board.
- **Interim analysis** (synonyms: unblinded analysis or comparative analysis) refers to an analysis that is conducted prior to the formal completion of a trial with the intention of comparing study arms with respect to efficacy or safety.
- **Interim data** refers to data collected at any time prior to formal completion of a trial.
- **Unblinded analysis** (synonym: comparative analysis) refers to an analysis that is conducted with known assignment of treatments. Interim analyses are often considered unblinded analyses since they require blinding of the treatment allocation to be broken.

Unifying Property of Adaptive Trial Designs

While there are countless variations of adaptive trial designs, the key unifying property of all adaptive trial designs includes the use of accumulating interim data based on pre-specified plans to adapt the designs of an ongoing trial [4]. Interim data refers to the data collected at any time prior to formal completion of a trial that is referenced to the target or maximum sample size or number of events of the trial. The use of interim data in adaptive trial designs often constitutes an analysis that is intended to compare study arms with respect to efficacy or safety (an interim analysis) [5]. Interim analyses have previously been referred to as comparative analyses or unblinded analyses, as interim analyses often entail breaking of treatment groups and comparison of study groups for efficacy [6]. The use of interim data may not always involve an unblinded interim analysis; for example, a blinded analysis of number of total events observed at the time of interim assessment could be used to re-estimate the sample size in blinded sample size re-assessment procedures [7].

The general flow of an adaptive trial design planning process can be seen in Figure 3.1. It is a common misconception that adaptive trial designs allow decisions to be made based on an ad hoc basis. Adaptive trials are conducted with pre-specified plans that are established before interim data are used for potential modifications of the trial, unlike conventional clinical trials where unplanned ad hoc modifications can be more common [4]. Often

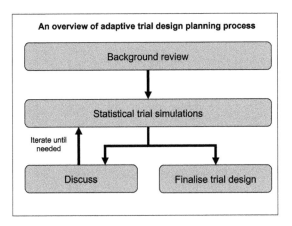

An overview of adaptive trial design planning process

Figure 3.1 An overview of general adaptive trial design planning process.

The general flow of adaptive trial design planning process starts with a background review for relevant clinical context and historical data or trial data that can be used as informed guesses to come up with realistic trial simulation scenarios. This is followed by an iterative cycle of trial simulations with clinical trial investigators before finalising the trial design.

guided by trial simulations, prospective planning requires specification of how the interim data will be used, who will perform the analyses, who will review the interim data, and other details that pertain to the statistical validity and integrity of the trial. As part of the interim analyses plan, details on the endpoint, statistical analyses, decision rules (e.g., early stopping if the calculated p-value < 0.01), timing and frequency of interim analyses [3, 8].

General conduct of clinical trials with adaptive trial designs can be seen in Figure 3.2. As similar to the conventional trials, adaptive trials will start enrolling after the trial protocol is finalised and approved for ethics and regulatory approval. In every adaptive trial, there is so-called burn-in period, where a pre-specified number of patients or number of events has been recruited or observed before the first interim analysis (or blinded assessment) is conducted. After one or more interim analyses, the trial may continue with or without adaptations, until the trial is ready to terminate due to the target sample size or number of events being reached, or when stopping rules are met.

It should be noted that trial monitoring for reasons other than potential trial design modifications is a routine practice, regardless of the design (adaptive or conventional). For instance, the primary responsibilities of the Data and Safety Monitoring Board (DSMB) often include review of accumulated trial data for safety, study conduct, and progress. Regardless of the design, adverse monitoring is an ethical standard for clinical trial research. In terms of study conduct and progress, data on recruitment, retention, and other performance metrics are often monitored to ensure successful trial completion in a timely manner [9]. Since patient recruitment and retention are two common reasons for trial failure, adequacy of goals and milestones for recruitment and retention at various trial sites will often be monitored [9].

Advantages and Limitations of Adaptive Trial Designs

Adaptive trial designs can have important advantages over conventional fixed sample trial designs, since by design, they allow the trial to adjust to information that was not available at the design stage [6]. Statistical efficiency is perhaps the most common advantage of adaptive trial designs. In comparison to conventional (non-adaptive) trials, the use of interim analyses that allow early stopping can lower the expected sample size or trial duration; designs that allow for modifications of the sample size can also improve the statistical power

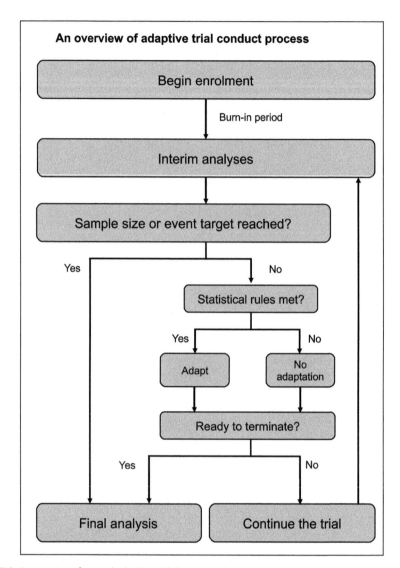

Figure 3.2 An overview of general adaptive trial design conduct.
The conduct of adaptive clinical trials starts with a burn-in period before the first interim analysis is conducted. After one or more interim analyses, the trial may continue with or without making adaptations. If decision rules are not met, the trial will continue until the next scheduled interim analysis or may be finished without making any adaptations.

to detect a true treatment effect [7]. The features of adaptive trial designs can provide ethical advantages over conventional designs. When the interim data show that the trial is unlikely to demonstrate effectiveness, stopping the trial early can reduce the number of patients who are exposed to ineffective experimental interventions and even allow for evaluation of other alternative interventions that may be more promising. It has been suggested that in trials that preferentially adapt the allocation ratio in favour of the treatment arm(s) with more favourable interim analysis results, both patients and physicians may be more likely to participate in the clinical trial [10].

There are limitations to adaptive trial designs. In comparison to conventional designs, adaptive trial designs offer more flexibility, but such flexibility will include statistical complexity. For fixed sample designs, there are well-established techniques for sample size calculations [11]. Sample size requirements for many conventional trials can be determined using a mathematical formula (i.e., a closed-form expression). Statistical planning of conventional trials is relatively straightforward and arguably easier than adaptive trial designs. For adaptive trial designs, it is often not possible to derive closed-form expressions, so evaluation of statistical properties (operating characteristics), such as expected sample size, type I error rate, and statistical power, requires the use of trial simulations [3, 12]. Often these simulation methods are not readily available and require methodological development. Statistical planning of adaptive trial designs can thus require more effort and time than conventional designs.

The use of adaptive trial designs can be logistically and operationally challenging. The use of interim analysis requires high-quality data to be available in a timely manner, so this can put more demands on the trial sites and their staff who will be performing the day-to-day trial activities [13]. Maintaining blinding, firewall of data, and information flow can be difficult throughout adaptive trial designs [6, 14]. It could be that operational partners may not have experience conducting adaptive clinical trials, and it can be difficult to anticipate the increased operational demands with the trial sites and staff. They may require additional training and education to meet the operational demands for an adaptive clinical trial.

Principles of Adaptive Trial Designs

A Priori Evaluation of Statistical Properties

The trial planning of adaptive trial designs often requires the use of statistical simulations. A priori evaluation of statistical properties, such as demonstration of expected type I error rate control, is a requirement for regulatory agencies such as the U.S. Food and Drug Administration for many of the registrational trials (trials conducted to support the filing of an application for regulatory approval) [15, 16]. Control of type I error rate is also a common constraint for non-registrational trials mandated by ethics boards or funding agencies. Many of the more complex trials with multiple adaptations planned will usually have several goals in addition to meeting the type I error rate constraint, so evaluation of their statistical properties can often be more multi-faceted. In addition to the evaluation of sample size, type I error rate, and power, other performance characteristics such as stopping probabilities at each interim analysis, estimated treatment effects, number of patients assigned to an inferior treatment, and more will often be evaluated using trial simulations.

Pre-specified plans for adaptive trial designs should be clearly outlined in study documents. Information on adaptive trial design could be outlined in the trial protocol or in the DSMB charter or statistical analysis plans, which could be separate documents from the main protocol documents. Good documentation practice (who saw what, when and why, and how) is often required, following the principle of 'if it isn't written down, then it didn't happen'.

Simulation-Guided Trial Planning

Trial planning is a complex process that requires considerations of several factors. Every clinical trial deserves a thorough investigation and consideration of the pros and cons using clinical trial simulations before selecting a specific design option and enrolling patients into the trial. It is important to recognise that an efficient trial design for one trial can be inefficient for another, and there is no such thing as a free lunch, meaning it is not possible to achieve something desirable without having to pay for it in some way [17]. Each design option will likely have trade-offs in terms of potential advantages and disadvantages. Therefore, a simulation-guided design process that will consider multiple design candidates during the planning stage to weigh the efficiencies of different design will be important [3, 18].

Proper Operational Oversight and Management

Adaptive trial designs can often pose operational complexities. As stated previously, conducting interim analyses requires access to high-quality data to be available in a timely manner. This will require timely data cleaning and transfer processes. It is generally not required for completely clean datasets with observations of all outcomes, but the minimal dataset to carry out interim analyses requires data on the endpoint (e.g., primary endpoint) and/or covariates that are pre-specified in the interim statistical analysis plan. Implementing pre-planned adaptations may not always be straightforward. For instance, knowledge of accumulating data or interim analysis results can affect the conduct of the trial due to the altered behaviours of the sponsors, investigators, trial staff, and/or participants (operational bias) [13, 15]. To mitigate operational bias, it is recommended that access to interim analysis results be limited to those personnel who are independent of the trial conduct and management [5]. No sponsors should have access to interim data. Independent oversights in forms of an independent statistical analysis centre and independent DSMB are important for adaptive clinical trials. Such independent oversight can help minimise operational bias and maintain scientific credibility.

There are adaptive trial designs where maintaining confidentiality can be difficult. For instance, for an adaptive trial that increases the sample size, it may not be possible to prevent such information from being known; this could indicate to investigators that there was lower treatment effects observed at an interim analysis, and this could possibly slow down recruitment after the adaptation [16]. Instead of notifying the trial sites that target sample size has been increased, it could be communicated that target enrolment has not been reached.

Summary

Adaptive trial designs offer pre-planned opportunities to modify aspects of an ongoing trial based on accumulating trial data. The use of interim data and pre-specified plans for potential adaptations is the key unifying property of adaptive trial designs and the key distinction from conventional trial designs. While the decisions for potential adaptations are made during the trial based on interim data, the flexibilities in adaptive trial designs are established and are outlined in the study documents, often before any patient is recruited into the trial. Adaptive trial designs offer more flexibility in comparison to conventional designs, but they do come with additional complexity.

References

1. Dimairo M, Pallmann P, Wason J, et al. The Adaptive Designs CONSORT Extension (ACE) statement: a checklist with explanation and elaboration guideline for reporting randomised trials that use an adaptive design. *BMJ*. 2020;**369**:m115.

2. Dimairo M, Pallmann P, Wason J, et al. The adaptive designs CONSORT extension (ACE) statement: a checklist with explanation and elaboration guideline for reporting randomised trials that use an adaptive design. *Trials*. 2020;**21**(1):528.

3. Thorlund K, Haggstrom J, Park JJ, Mills EJ. Key design considerations for adaptive clinical trials: a primer for clinicians. *BMJ*. 2018;**360**:k698.

4. Pallmann P, Bedding AW, Choodari-Oskooei B, et al. Adaptive designs in clinical trials: why use them, and how to run and report them. *BMC Med*. 2018;**16**(1):29.

5. ICH Harmonised Tripartite Guideline. Statistical principles for clinical trials. International Conference on Harmonisation E9 Expert Working Group. *Stat Med*. 1999;**18**(15):1905–42.

6. U.S. Food and Drug Administration. *The Establishment and Operation of Clinical Trial Data Monitoring Committees for Clinical Trial Sponsors*. United States Department of Health and Human Services; 2006.

7. Bhatt DL, Mehta C. Adaptive designs for clinical trials. *N Engl J Med*. 2016;**375**(1):65–74.

8. Park JJ, Thorlund K, Mills EJ. Critical concepts in adaptive clinical trials. *Clin Epidemiol*. 2018;**10**:343–51.

9. Fogel DB. Factors associated with clinical trials that fail and opportunities for improving the likelihood of success: a review. *Contemp Clin Trials Commun*. 2018;**11**:156–64.

10. Tehranisa JS, Meurer WJ. Can response-adaptive randomization increase participation in acute stroke trials? *Stroke*. 2014;**45**(7):2131–3.

11. Florey CD. Sample size for beginners. *BMJ*. 1993;**306**(6886):1181–4.

12. Hummel J, Wang S, Kirkpatrick J. Using simulation to optimize adaptive trial designs: applications in learning and confirmatory phase trials. *Clin Invest*. 2015;**5**(4):401–13.

13. Detry MA, Lewis RJ, Broglio KR, Standards for the design, conduct, and evaluation of adaptive randomized clinical trials. Patient-Centered Outcomes Research Institute (PCORI); 2012.

14. Sanchez-Kam M, Gallo P, Loewy J, et al. A practical guide to data monitoring committees in adaptive trials. *Ther Innov Regul Sci*. 2014;**48**(3):316–26.

15. U.S. Food and Drug Administration. *Adaptive Designs for Medical Device Clinical Studies Guidance for Industry and Food and Drug Administration Staff*. United States Department of Health and Human Services; 2016.

16. United States Department of Health and Human Services, Food and Drug Administration. *Adaptive Designs for Clinical Trials of Drugs and Biologics. Guidance for Industry*. Center for Biologics Evaluation and Research (CBER); 2019.

17. Bauer P, Bretz F, Dragalin V, Konig F, Wassmer G. Twenty-five years of confirmatory adaptive designs: opportunities and pitfalls. *Stat Med*. 2016;**35**(3):325–47.

18. Burton A, Altman DG, Royston P, Holder RL. The design of simulation studies in medical statistics. *Stat Med*. 2006;**25**(24):4279–92.

Common Types of Adaptive Trial Designs

Chapter 4

Jay J. H. Park, J. Kyle Wathen, and Edward J. Mills

Key Points of This Chapter

This chapter discusses the common types of adaptive trial designs and their motivations and challenges. The key points of this chapter are:

- Sequential designs that use interim analyses to allow for early stopping are the most common type of adaptive trial designs. Sequential designs are often used with other types of adaptive trial designs.

- Other common types of adaptive trial designs include sample size re-assessment that uses blinded or unblinded data for re-estimation of sample size during the trial; response adaptive randomisation that preferentially increases allocation ratio in favour of treatment arm based on interim trial data; adaptive enrichment design that allows for modification of patient eligibility criteria; and seamless design that combines two phases of clinical trial research into one trial.

- In comparison to conventional fixed trial designs, adaptive trial designs can offer more flexibility, but this can pose complexities that usually require more thorough and thoughtful planning in the design stage. Adaptive trial designs can result in notable efficiencies for the right questions, but this is not always the case. Trade-offs between different design options should be carefully considered.

Introduction

As discussed in the last chapter, we have learned that adaptive trial designs refer to a group of trial designs that offer pre-planned opportunities to modify aspects of an ongoing trial based on accumulating trial data [1, 2]. There are many countless variations of adaptive trial designs, but common design features targeted for adaptations include sample size, allocation ratios, and eligibility criteria [3]. Different types of adaptive trial designs are often referred to and grouped by their targeted area of potential modifications. As outlined in Table 4.1, common types of adaptive trial designs include but are not limited to *sequential design*; *sample size re-assessment minimisation*; *response adaptive randomisation*; *adaptive enrichment design*; and *seamless design* [3–5]. In this chapter, we discuss these common designs in detail and their motivations and challenges.

Table 4.1 Common types of adaptive trial designs
An overview of common types of adaptive trial designs is provided in this table.

Design types	Details
Sequential design	Refers to a group of designs that allows one or more interim analyses to be conducted to stop the trial early in a case of a two-arm trial, or a study arm in case of a multi-arm. Early stopping can be made based on either superiority and/or futility.
Sample size re-assessment	Allows target sample size or number of events to be re-estimated during the trial to ensure the desired statistical power.
Minimisation*	A common type of adaptive randomisation that adapts allocation based on pre-specified covariates to minimise imbalance of these prognostic factors between groups being compared.
Response adaptive randomisation	Allows allocation ratios to be preferentially adapted over time in favour of study arm(s) with more favourable interim results; also referred to as 'outcome' adaptive randomisation since patient outcome data are used to adapt the allocation.
Adaptive enrichment design	Allows for potential modification of trial eligibility to narrower group of patients who are more likely to benefit from assigned treatment.
Seamless design	Two phases of clinical trials are connected to allow for immediate continuation from one phase to the subsequent phase (e.g., seamless phase IIB/III design).

* Minimisation (the most common type of covariate adaptive randomisation) and response adaptive randomisation (also known as outcome adaptive randomisation) fall under the broad umbrella category of adaptive randomisation designs, where the allocation probabilities are adapted based on accruing information throughout the trial. In minimisation, allocation probabilities change based on the covariates observed, and response adaptive randomisation adapts the allocation probabilities based on the observed outcomes.

Common Types of Adaptive Trial Designs

Sequential Design

Sequential designs refer to a group of designs that allow for early stopping based on interim analyses [6, 7]. Interim analyses in this context would entail generating performance metrics on the effectiveness and not just monitoring the trial progress from the data that are being collected. In the case of a two-arm trial, early stopping applies to the entire trial; early stopping applies to a specific study arm in the case of a multi-arm trial (Figure 4.1). In sequential designs, a test statistic (e.g., a p-value) is calculated during an interim analysis, and if the test statistic meets a pre-specified threshold, the trial or that specific arm generally will stop [8]. If pre-specified thresholds are not met, the trial will continue as before.

If interim analysis shows promising results for a treatment, the allocation ratio can be modified to favour enrolment to that treatment. In adaptive enrichment, if interim analysis shows that a treatment has more promising results in one sub-group of patients, the study

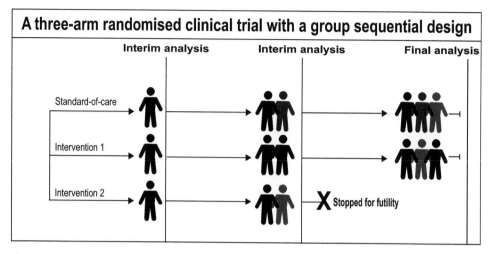

Figure 4.1 An illustration of a group sequential design.

Group sequential design: A three-arm randomised clinical trial with two interim analyses. In this example, Intervention 2 meets the futility threshold at the second interim analysis and is therefore dropped from the trial. This contrasts a typically used approach in a fixed sample trial design that would have only a single final analysis.

eligibility criteria can be modified to investigate the efficacy of the intervention in the that sub-group, with a sample size reassessment to ensure a sufficient sample size.

In sequential designs, early stopping can be made based on benefit (superiority), futility, and harm. Early stopping for superiority can be made if the interim data show that the intervention has sufficient evidence to conclude that it is effective. If the interim data show that a given intervention demonstrates lack of benefit or lack of sufficient activity, early stopping can be done for futility [9]. In other words, futility can declared when the intervention has demonstrated it has convincingly no benefit, or when it has a low chance of demonstrating eventual success even if more patients would be randomised to that intervention arm [9–11]. Criteria for stopping based on harm are often different from stopping criteria for superiority and harm in that it may not employ a formal statistical criterion [12]. Harm is often used as a synonym for patient safety and adverse events in the literature, but harm should refer to the totality of possible adverse events and other consequences of an intervention [13]. Monitoring of harm is important to enable appropriate management of adverse events, and documentation of trial-related adverse events is critical to inform clinical practice. The importance of monitoring for harm applies to conventional clinical trials as well as adaptive trial designs.

Sequential designs are useful for many instances because there is often substantial uncertainty in the likely treatment effects when a clinical trial is being designed. If the assumed treatment effect is an underestimation of the true treatment effect, the planned sample size may be larger than necessary. This is where interim analyses for superiority would be useful to lower the expected sample size of the trial. If the assumed treatment effect is an overestimation, that will result in the trial being underpowered to detect an effect that is clinically meaningful and worthy of changing in patient management. The required sample size could be considerably larger than the maximum sample size that is feasible to recruit. Since there will be low statistical power to detect a treatment effect in such case, futility interim analyses can be used as a way of cutting your losses early. Sequential designs can lower the expected sample size of the trial.

In the early literature on sequential methodology, continuous monitoring of the gradually accumulating data has been discussed, but it is generally more acceptable to use a 'group sequential' approach where a limited number of pre-planned interim analyses are conducted [14–17]. Repeated 'looks' at the accumulating data increases the false error rate in a clinical trial, so we usually need a safeguard against inflated false error risks. In case of early stopping for superiority, one can incorrectly declare that the intervention being evaluated is superior in an interim analysis, so repeated looks in this context can inflate the type I error rate. Stopping criteria for an superiority interim analysis are usually set stringently in anticipation of multiplicity (inflated type I error rate due to multiple testing) and to ensure that the overall type I error rate of the trial does not exceed the desired alpha (e.g., 0.05) [8]. In early stopping for futility, there is no option to stop early and declare that the intervention is superior, so this does not inflate the type I error rate. Futility interim analyses can, however, lower the statistical power, as it can falsely stop enrolment early. Similar to stopping criteria for superiority interim analyses, stringent criteria for futility are used, and the sample size is usually increased modestly to compensate for the reduced statistical power.

Sequential designs are the most common type of adaptive trial design [3–5]. Sequential designs are often used with other adaptive trial design features, so in a single trial, multiple areas of adaptations may be pre-specified and be adopted [18]. For instance, a clinical trial with sequential design may be used with sample size re-assessment with sample size target being increased to ensure the statistical power can be maintained at the desired level [5]. Bhatt and Mehta have defined group sequential designs used with sample size re-assessment, where the target sample size or number of events can be re-calculated during the trial as 'adaptive group sequential designs', whereas group sequential designs where the maximum sample size or events cannot be changed as 'classic group sequential designs' [5].

Metrics Used for Stopping Rules

Stopping boundaries or rules are commonly based on the frequentist metrics of p-value and conditional power and Bayesian metrics of posterior probability and predictive probability [3, 10, 19]. As discussed in Chapter 1, p-value informally refers to the probability of observing a test statistic as extreme or more extreme as one did assuming the null hypothesis. Conditional power (also referred to as stochastic curtailment) refers to a probability that the final result will be significant at some future sample size, given the data obtained up to the time of the interim look and assuming a specific value of treatment effects [20]. For the assumption of specific value of treatment effects, it is common to use the treatment effects that are observed in the interim analysis, or to retain the original treatment effect size that was assumed in the design stage. In a Bayesian framework, a common metric that is used for decision making is the posterior probability of superiority that can be defined as the probability of the treatment being superior to the control. This metric is often used for interim monitoring [10]. In comparison to p-values, probability of superiority or other probability-based metrics may be less prone to misinterpretation [21]. Bayesian predictive probability (also referred to as predictive power) refers to a probability of eventual success at the future sample size given the current data and assumed prior distributions [10, 11]. In contrast to conditional power that is often criticised for assuming the unknown treatment parameter to be fixed at a specific value, Bayesian predictive probability averages the probability of eventual success over the variability of the treatment effect parameter estimates [10, 11].

Stopping Rules

When using sequential design, researchers need to decide how error rates should be controlled and what statistical metrics will be used. There are multiple possible stopping rules that can be based on either frequentist or Bayesian metrics [14]. In anticipation of multiplicity due to repeated testing, more stringent statistical criteria are often used at interim analyses or in general than fixed sample trial designs. The amount of information (data) at a given interim analysis divided by the total information is referred to as the 'information fraction' [22]. For a clinical trial that has pre-specified a target sample size, the sample size available at the time of interim analysis would be used to calculate its information fraction. For an event-driven trial that has pre-specified a target number of events, the information fraction is calculated with the number of events available at the interim analysis. In most cases, stopping rules are a function of information fraction.

Frequentist Stopping Rules

Table 4.2 shows three group sequential tests that are commonly used for superiority interim analyses: Pocock [6], O'Brien–Fleming [23], and Haybittle–Peto [24, 25] tests. These efficacy boundaries in these group sequential tests are based on Z statistics that correspond

Table 4.2 O'Brien–Fleming, Haybittle–Peto, and Pocock stopping boundaries for superiority interim analyses This table shows the nominal significance levels of three common stopping boundaries used in group sequential designs for an overall type I error rate of 0.05 at interim analysis frequency of 1, 2, and 3.

Analysis number	Information fraction	Significance level: alpha (α)		
		Pocock	O'Brien–Fleming	Haybittle–Peto
Number of statistical analyses: 2				
1st interim analysis	0.50	0.0294	0.0054	0.0020
Final (2nd) analysis	1.00	0.0294	0.0492	0.0500
Number of statistical analyses: 3				
1st interim analysis	0.33	0.0221	0.0006	0.0010
2nd interim analysis	0.67	0.0221	0.0151	0.0010
Final (3rd) analysis	1.00	0.0221	0.0471	0.0500
Number of statistical analyses: 4				
1st interim analysis	0.25	0.0182	0.00005	0.00100
2nd interim analysis	0.50	0.0182	0.0039	0.00100
3rd interim analysis	0.75	0.0182	0.0184	0.00100
Final (4th) analysis	1.00	0.0182	0.0412	0.0500

to p-values (alpha) that the interim analysis needs to demonstrate for the trial to stop early for superiority. Table 4.2 shows the significance values for equally spaced-out analyses ranging from 2, 3, and 4 for an overall type I error rate of 0.05. For instance, when there are two analyses with one interim analysis planned at an information fraction of 0.50. Between these different approaches, the distribution of the overall significance ('alpha spent') at each analysis is different. For instance, the Pocock test maintains the identical significance levels needed to reject the null hypothesis at each of the analyses [6]. This is similar to the most conservative option in the Bonferroni correction, where the overall alpha is simply divided by the number of the planned analyses. The O'Brien–Fleming and Haybittle–Peto tests both use much more stringent stopping criteria at interim analyses and maintain a closer or exact significance level at the final analysis [23–25].

Out of the three tests, the Pocock test provides the best chance of early termination, but this results in having the worst chance of rejecting the null hypothesis at the final analysis. Since the final analysis could show a statistically significant result if interim analyses would not have been adopted, the Pocock test is often viewed unfavourably. The Haybittle–Peto test is also sometimes viewed unfavourably because stopping early becomes very unlikely due to its stringent significance levels used at interim analyses. However, an advantage with the Haybittle–Peto test is that a full alpha (e.g., 0.05) can be maintained for the final analysis.

There are drawbacks to group sequential tests. They require equal spacing between scheduled analyses with respect to the maximum sample size or number of events and the number of interim analyses that must be defined a priori. It is often not always feasible to conduct an interim analysis exactly at a specific fraction of the planned total sample size or number of events. To allow for flexibility in how many interim analyses and when they can be conducted, alpha spending function is often used [26]. Alpha spending allows the timing of interim analyses to be flexible; here, the stopping criteria for superiority is calculated as a function of the information fraction at the time of interim analysis [27]. The Lan–DeMets spending function and the Kim–DeMets spending function are common approaches to alpha spending functions [28, 29]. Lan–DeMets in 1983 showed that alpha spending functions that can approximate the stopping boundaries of O'Brien–Fleming test or Pocock test to control the overall type I error rate [28].

In the case of a two-arm trial, it is possible to stop the trial early for reasons other than superiority (beneficial effect). The intervention being evaluated could clearly lack clinical benefit or have little to no chance of demonstrating clinical benefit even if more patients were recruited into the trial. It is important during trial monitoring to ask the question, 'Given the current results of the trial, what is the probability that the eventual conclusions will change if the trial goes through as originally planned?' [30]. Conditional power (stochastic curtailment) is a useful tool for trial monitoring, particularly for futility monitoring since it allows one to ask such a question [30]. Conditional power allows for the calculation of the probability of rejecting the null hypothesis at the end of the trial given the data collected thus far, assuming the point estimate of the treatment effects observed at the interim analysis, or the original effect size assumed in the design stage. Analogous to alpha spending functions, there are beta spending functions that control for beta that gets 'spent' at each futility interim analysis to control for the type II error rate [31]. Beta spending functions can help monitor and control the stage-wise and overall power (type II error rate control) that can be induced by futility interim analyses [31].

Bayesian Stopping Rules

Discussion thus far has largely focused on stopping rules based on frequentist metrics that have dominated the literature on sequential methodology early on. With increasing computational capabilities for statistical models, the use of Bayesian statistics has been increasing in clinical trial research [19, 32]. In the context of sequential designs and other adaptive trial designs, a Bayesian paradigm can afford the flexibility to update uncertainties and carry them into the future in the presence of the interim trial data [19]. Bayesian statistics are often used as a tool for frequentist clinical trials in the sense that even these clinical trials with Bayesian stopping rules are often required to meet the type I error rate constraint (e.g., 5.0% type I error rate). Clinical trial simulation is performed under the null effect scenario that assumes that the treatment has a null effect (no treatment effect) to estimate the expected type I error rate of the trial design. Even though Bayesian stopping rules are used, they will often be required to demonstrate the same frequentist statistical constraints as other clinical trials that use frequentist stopping rules. Bayesian stopping rules often can demonstrate more favourable frequentist operating characteristics such as type I error rate and statistical power than frequentist stopping rules [19]. One should always consider how the choice of the prior distribution and the effects it will have on the trial results when a Bayesian approach is utilised.

Stopping rules can be based on metrics of posterior and predictive probabilities. Let us consider a trial evaluating a treatment that aims to reduce mortality at 28 days. The trial could be designed to detect some magnitude of treatment effect summarised by an odds ratio (OR). With an OR that is less than 1 representing a more favourable treatment effect, the superiority threshold for early stopping could be defined as the 97.5% posterior probability of an OR being less than 1. If an interim analysis shows a posterior probability that is greater than 97.5%, this Bayesian sequential trial would stop enrolment early and declare that the treatment arm is superior to the control. Otherwise, the trial would continue to the next interim analysis. The 97.5% threshold here is somewhat arbitrary, as such a threshold is often calibrated using trial simulations to meet the type I error constraint while maximising other operating characteristics such as statistical power and sample size. Similarly, futility thresholds can be defined using posterior probability. As the superiority threshold example, the futility threshold could be defined 10% posterior probability of an OR being less than 1, where if less than 10% posterior probability is observed at an interim analysis, the trial could stop early based on futility reasoning. Again, the specific futility threshold here is arbitrary and mentioned for an illustrative purpose.

As an alternative to conditional power, the use of Bayesian predictive probability of success and predictive power was first proposed by Spiegelhalter and colleagues in 1986 for trial monitoring [33]. Like conditional power, Bayesian predictive probability represents the probability of eventual success if more patients would be enrolled given the current data and assumed prior distribution. Bayesian predictive probability has a key distinction to conditional power in that it does not need to assume a specific fixed value of treatment effect [10, 11]. Bayesian predictive probability moves away from such strong assumptions, and it averages over a distribution of potential treatment effects instead [10, 11]. The Bayesian predictive probability is a useful tool for trial monitoring. It can be used as stopping criteria for futility and superiority. Predictive probability has been used as a superiority threshold in phase II settings, where the superiority threshold was based on an eventual success in a phase III confirmatory trial [34, 35].

Common Concerns for Stopping Early

Common concerns that exist in sequential designs include false error rate associated with stopping and bias in the estimate of the treatment effect. We have already discussed extensively how false error rate can be controlled for in sequential designs. For biased estimation, stopping early for superiority can introduce some positive bias and result in an overestimation of the treatment effect; whereas futility can introduce negative bias resulting in an underestimated treatment effect [36]. However, the magnitude of bias for early stopping is generally small, especially if the size of the burn-in (sample size at the first interim analysis) is adequately large [36, 37]. Ethical and efficiency considerations should outweigh the concerns for bias associated with sequential designs [37].

Sample Size Re-Assessment

Sample size calculations are done to achieve a specific power that depends on the true effect size and variability of the endpoint [38]. Appropriate sample size calculations are dependent on correct assumptions of design parameters such as variance for continuous endpoints and event rates for binary endpoints. These assumptions are often based on findings from historical studies, but making such assumptions based on previous studies can have limitations. Between historical studies, even if they are from the same clinical development program, there can be important differences. As sample size requirements generally increase from early phase to later phase trials, additional trial sites from different geographic settings may be added. There are also temporal variabilities that exist, so it is difficult to determine the required sample size accurately.

When a trial fails to meet its pre-specified endpoints under such a circumstance, simply enrolling more patients is not a valid option since the control of type I error rate can no longer be guaranteed if it is done on an ad hoc basis [39]. Sample size re-assessment is a type of adaptive trial design that has been developed to mitigate risks for false-negative findings due to trials being under powered (Figure 4.2). Sample size re-assessment refers to an adaptive

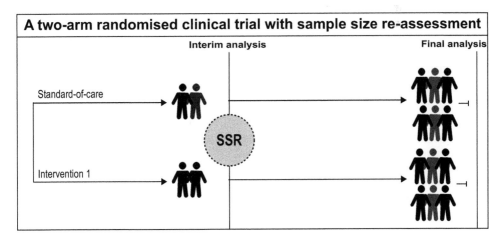

Figure 4.2 An illustration of sample size re-assessment design.

Sample size re-assessment: A two-arm randomised clinical trial with one interim analysis. In this example, an unblinded interim analysis is conducted to increase the final sample size target to ensure that the trial is adequately powered.

SSR = sample size re-assessment

trial design that allows for adjustment of sample size to ensure desired statistical power [7]. These designs can broadly be classified into two groups: (1) blinded and (2) unblinded sample size re-assessments [5]. Blinded sample size re-assessment procedure involves estimation of the variance or the overall event rate of the primary endpoint from blinded interim data, where the observations from both groups are pooled without revealing the data at the level of the individual study arm [40]. Unblinded sample size re-assessment procedure, on the other hand, involves re-assessment of sample size based on unblinded interim treatment effect estimates [5]. Conditional power or Bayesian predictive power can be used to determine the sample size that is required to ensure sufficient statistical power [10, 11].

There are challenges with sample size re-assessment methods, particularly the unblinded procedure. For the unblinded re-assessment procedure, the interim estimate of the treatment effect can be misleading if it is based on small partial data [5]. The unblinded re-assessment procedure will require adjustments when calculating point estimates and confidence intervals to preserve the type I error rate and to avoid bias in estimation [41]. Simple procedures for blinded sample size re-assessment generally do not affect the type I error rate [42]. However, blinded and unblinded sample size re-assessment procedures will require strict firewalls to prevent leakage of information about decisions. Knowledge of the change in the sample size target is potentially a concern for operational bias, where the investigators' behaviour may change as a result [5].

Adaptive Randomisation

In clinical trials with adaptive randomisation designs, allocation probabilities are adapted based on accruing information during the trial [43]. Covariate adaptive randomisation and response adaptive randomisation are two common types of randomisation procedures that fall under the umbrella of adaptive randomisation [43]. In covariate adaptive randomisation, allocation ratio is adjusted based on the baseline prognostic values of patients who had already been randomised generally to achieve better balance of pre-specified prognostic factors [43, 44]. Response adaptive randomisation, also referred to as outcome adaptive randomisation, uses interim data to adapt the allocation ratio in favour of the study arm that is performing better [45]. In this section, we introduce minimisation, the most common covariate adaptive randomisation design, as well as response adaptive randomisation methods in more detail.

Minimisation

Minimisation is a procedure that adapts allocation to minimise imbalance of pre-specified prognostic factors between groups being compared in a clinical trial. The treatment allocation of the new patient enrolling into the trial is determined based on the characteristics of the patients already enrolled. With minimisation, the degree of imbalance that would occur if a new patient was assigned to either treatment groups is calculated and then compared before determining their allocation into the trial.

Suppose that we are running a two-arm clinical trial where we wish to balance patients with respect to three factors: age (younger than 50 vs. 50 or order), race (white vs. non-white), and sex (male vs. female). There are 60 patients who are already enrolled in the trial with the baseline characteristics outlined in Table 4.3, and the new patient to enter our trial is a 40-year-old white male. With minimisation, the degree of imbalance over all pre-specified prognostic factors would be summed and then compared to determine the allocation of the next patient.

Table 4.3 A hypothetical distribution of baseline characteristics after 60 patients for minimisation
A hypothetical distribution of baseline characteristics shown here to illustrate the concept of minimisation.

Factor	Levels	Number of patients on Treatment A (n = 30)	Number of patients on Treatment B (n = 30)	Next patient
Age	<50 years	20	19	*
	≥50 years	10	11	
Race	White	10	9	*
	Non-white	20	21	
Sex	Male	14	15	*
	Female	16	15	

In this illustrative example of minimisation, if this 40-year-old white male patient is randomised to Treatment A, the imbalance would increase in age (<50 years old) and race (white) and decrease in sex (male):

$$= (20 + 1) - 19 \text{ for Age} + (10 + 1) - 9 \text{ for Race} + (14 + 1) - 15 \text{ for Sex}$$
$$= 2 \, (\text{Age}) + 2 \, (\text{Race}) - 0 \, (\text{Sex}) = 4.$$

If this patient is randomised to Treatment B, the imbalance would conversely decrease in age and race and increase in sex, but since the overall imbalance would decrease:

$$= 20 - (19 + 1) \text{ for Age} + 10 - (9 + 1) \text{ for Race} + 14 - (15 + 1) \text{ for Sex}$$
$$= 0 \, (\text{Age}) + 0 \, (\text{Race}) - 2 \, (\text{Sex}) = 2.$$

Now that we have determined that allocating this 40-year-old white male patient to Treatment B would decrease overall imbalance, the minimisation method would adapt the allocation ratio in favour of Treatment B. There are two different types of minimisation procedures. The deterministic minimisation procedure would just simply allocate the patient to Treatment B [46–48]. The stochastic minimisation procedure would use a weighted randomisation that would give higher chance (e.g., 80%) of the patient being randomised to Treatment B [48, 49]. While the stochastic minimisation still could result in this patient being randomly allocated to Treatment A (e.g., 20%) where the overall imbalance is between groups, the random element makes the stochastic minimisation more preferable than the deterministic minimisation that is not based on random chance. In both types of minimisation procedures, the process is repeated for each subsequent patient. When there are no imbalances across all pre-specified prognostic factors, the subsequent randomisation would be made using simple randomisation [48].

Minimisation shares similarities to stratified randomisation. Both randomisation techniques aim to achieve covariate balance of one or more prognostic factors that can be measured at baseline between different groups being compared in a clinical trial. They both require prognostic factors to be identified before the trial starts. Stratified randomisation may not be effective when several variables are used, especially in small trials [50]. As minimisation can handle more prognostic variables, it has been argued that minimisation is superior to stratified randomisation [50]. However, if unimportant prognostic factors are chosen, minimisation may result in a balance that is not relevant for statistical inference. There are concerns over the validity of minimisation since the allocation procedure is wholly or partly dependent on known baseline factors, so the theoretical properties of achieving balance of both known and unknown factors are not clear [51]. Minimisation also can raise practical challenges. For instance, in stratified randomisation, the randomisation lists for different strata are produced before the trial starts. However, as outlined above, minimisation is a dynamic method that generates the randomisation during participant recruitment based on the previous allocations. Minimisation can make allocation concealment more difficult, so a secure allocation system overseen by an independent statistician is usually used [52]. This therefore can raise complexity and even the cost of clinical trial research when compared to stratified randomisation and other static randomisation procedures [52].

Response Adaptive Randomisation

Randomisation is an important tool that can help establish the highest level of evidence on the effectiveness of new interventions. The importance of randomisation in clinical research is generally widely accepted among the medical community, but there are challenges and perceived barriers associated with randomisation. Even in the presence of equipoise, clinicians often perceive randomisation as being uncomfortable and potentially conflicting with patient care [53]. Patients' willingness to participate in randomised clinical trials can also vary greatly [54]. Response adaptive randomisation has gained popularity recently, albeit controversial and polarising, to promote randomisation as being more comfortable [53, 55].

Response adaptive randomisation is a type of adaptive trial design in which allocation ratios are preferentially adapted in favour of study arm(s) based on interim results [56–58] (Figure 4.3). In contrast to minimisation and other types of covariate adaptive randomisation designs, response adaptive randomisation uses past treatment assignments and patient responses to adapt the allocation probability for future patients being enrolled. Since response adaptive randomisation uses outcome data, it is sometimes referred to as *outcome adaptive randomisation* [57, 58]. Rather than randomising patients at a fixed allocation ratio (e.g., 1:1 allocation), response adaptive randomisation is motivated by the idea that more patients could be randomised to the superior treatment and so minimise the number of treatment failures. Response adaptive randomisation has ethically appealing properties [59]. Some even have argued that it could be an effective strategy to improve physician participation and patient recruitment [60, 61].

There are many approaches to response adaptive randomisation. Let us consider an example of a two-arm Bayesian clinical trial for a binary response rate. The allocation ratio here can be adapted based on posterior probabilities of each study arm being better than the other. If the probability of Treatment A being better than the control is 0.75, then there is a 0.25 probability that the control is better than Treatment A. The original version of response adaptive randomisation that was introduced by Thompson would simply adapt the allocation ratios for Treatment A and the control as 0.75 and 0.25, respectively [62]. Since it is possible that the higher response rate observed in Treatment A is due to random variation, especially when there is a small sample size, it is recommended to have an adequate period of burn-in to allow a fixed number of patients to be randomised before adapting the allocation ratios. Additionally, it is often necessary to 'temper' the adaptive randomisation algorithm to avoid temporal biases that can result in a larger number of patients actually being assigned to the inferior treatment arm. It is common to add a square

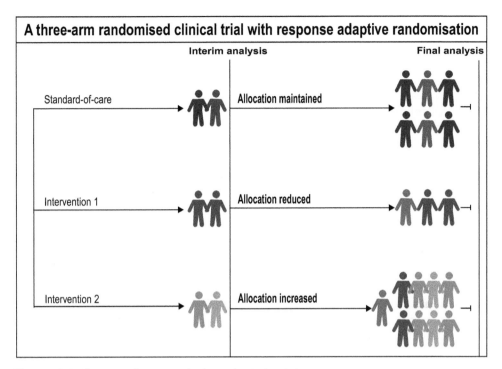

Figure 4.3 An illustration of response adaptive randomisation design.

Response adaptive randomisation: In this three-arm randomised clinical trial, response adaptive randomisation is used to increase allocation to Intervention 2 and to decrease allocation to Intervention 1 while maintaining allocation to the common control group. In the end, more patients end up receiving the favourable intervention.

root term in the calculation of allocation ratios to temper the adaptive randomisation algorithm [57]. For the response rates of 0.75 and 0.25 mentioned above, adding a square root term (power to 1/2) would result in allocation ratios of 0.63 and 0.37 that are higher than the Thompson example [57]. There are many other variations of how response adaptive randomisation can be calculated.

Allocation ratio for Treatment A:

$$= \text{Prob } (A > \text{Control})^{1/2} / [(\text{Prob of } A > \text{Control})^{1/2} + (\text{Prob of Control} > A)^{1/2}]$$
$$= (0.75^{1/2}) / [(0.75^{1/2}) + (0.25^{1/2})]$$
$$= (0.87) / [0.87 + 0.50]$$
$$= 0.63.$$

Allocation ratio for Control:

$$= \text{Prob } (\text{Control} > A)^{1/2} / [(\text{Prob of Control} > A)^{1/2} + (\text{Prob of } A > \text{Control})^{1/2}]$$
$$= (0.25^{1/2}) / [(0.25^{1/2}) + (0.75^{1/2})]$$
$$= (0.50) / [0.50 + 0.87]$$
$$= 0.37.$$

Response adaptive randomisation creates unequal balance of patients. Recall that in the first chapter we discussed that the block randomisation technique maximises statistical power by achieving equal balance in number of patients assigned to different study groups. If maximising statistical power is a primary concern when designing a two-arm trial, response adaptive randomisation perhaps should be avoided. Response adaptive random-isation can create inferential problems that may decrease benefits to patients enrolled in the trial as well as future patients [57]. For instance, it has been shown that response adaptive randomisation could result in a biased estimate of treatment effect and high probability of sample size imbalance in the wrong direction, where more patients end up being assigned to the inferior treatment [57].

The use of response adaptive randomisation in a two-arm trial setting deserves separate discussion from its use in a multi-arm setting. The proponents of response adaptive randomisation have argued that its polarising statistical properties in two-arm trials cannot be generalised to multi-arm trial settings [56]. Multi-arm trials are defined by clinical trials that have three or more study groups, but unlike two-arm trials, there can be numerous forms of trial comparisons [63]. If we consider a trial with three treatment groups (A, B, and C), possible comparisons include: (1) a common control comparison: A vs. C and B vs. C; (2) a global test that compares all at once: A vs. B vs. C; and (3) all pairwise comparisons: A vs. B, A vs. C, and B vs. C.

When there is a common control group, the trial involves multiple pairwise compari-sons to test more than once whether a given treatment is better than the control. Since the control comparisons are the primary focus, having too few patients in the control group can be problematic for statistical power [64]. It would even be beneficial to allocate more participants to the control [64]. Instead of applying the adaptive randomisation to the control group, maintaining a fixed allocation to the control group while adapting the allocation ratios between experimental interventions may be useful [56, 58]. When some intervention arms are terminated early, the sample size saved could be allocated to remain-ing arms [58]. For multi-arm trials where the primary comparison of interest involves a global test or all pairwise comparisons, the role of response adaptive randomisation is less certain [58]. It is recommended to have an adequate burn-in period, tempered adaptive allocation, and potentially minimum allocation to be maintained [58].

If one wishes to use response adaptive randomisation, the pros and cons of different adaptive randomisation algorithms should be carefully and thoroughly evaluated in the design stage using simulations. If it is believed that decreasing allocation to the control arm could improve recruitment and patient participation, using an unequal, fixed randomisa-tion (e.g., 2:1) could be considered in the design stage. In addition to statistical challenges, response adaptive randomisation can often raise operational complexities [65]. There have been multiple simulation studies that have examined statistical challenges and benefits of response adaptive randomisation. However, to our knowledge, limited examination has been done to assess whether response adaptive randomisation can increase participation of patients and health care providers who may be wary of participating in clinical trials. According to a 2018 Cochrane systematic literature review that examined different ran-domised and quasi-randomised trials on methods to increase clinical trial recruitment, there are no randomised clinical trials that have examined the effect of response adaptive randomisation on clinical trial participation [66]. There is one cross-sectional survey that randomly assigned patients to a video describing a hypothetical trial with or without response adaptive randomisation, but this did not actually involve real patient recruitment into an actual clinical trial [61].

Adaptive Enrichment Design

With advancements in genomic sequencing, there has been increased emphasis towards precision medicine, particularly in oncology, that aims to develop medical interventions that target diseases based on their genetic make-up [67]. This has increased emphasis on biomarker-guided clinical trials including adaptive enrichment designs [3, 4, 68]. Adaptive enrichment designs allow for modification of trial eligibility criteria based on an interim analysis to restrict future enrolment to narrower groups of patients who might be more responsive to treatments [69, 70]. These designs often involve screening and identification of predictive biomarkers (e.g., genetic mutations) with a purpose of identifying patients with such characteristic who will benefit from new treatments.

There have been different variations of adaptive enrichment designs reported [69, 70]. As general approaches to adaptive enrichment designs, the trial would start with an all-comers population regardless of their biomarker status (Figure 4.4). The effectiveness of a given therapy would be evaluated to see if the treatment effects would differ between biomarker-positive and -negative groups. If it is shown that the biomarker-positive sub-population is more likely to benefit from the treatment, an adaptation would be made to the trial eligibility that the biomarker-negative group would either be excluded for further enrolment from the study altogether or be reduced. The biomarker-positive group would then be 'enriched' with

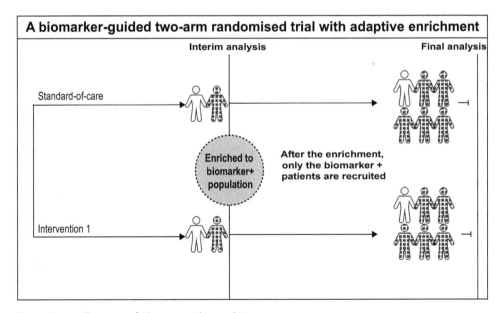

Figure 4.4 An illustration of adaptive enrichment design.

Adaptive enrichment design: In this two-arm randomised clinical trial, a biomarker-positive group of patients have more favourable results at the interim analysis. In accordance with the planned enrichment design, the trial is enriched when the study eligibility criteria are modified to investigate the efficacy of the intervention in the biomarker-positive group of patients.

larger sample size, so this approach has been referred to as 'sample enrichment' designs [69, 70]. In terms of statistical criteria for enrichment, conditional power or predictive power-based decision rules have been proposed [71, 72]. Here, the predictive probabilities of eventual success if the trial would be enriched to a pre-specified sub-population would be evaluated throughout the interim analysis to potentially allow for an enrichment decision.

There are challenges with adaptive enrichment designs [73]. Similar to other biomarker-guided trials, recruitment to a trial with an adaptive enrichment design relies on baseline information of biomarker status. This can raise operational and logistical complexities associated with timely handling and transport of biospecimens for biomarker assessment. There should not be long delay in time to ascertain biomarker status; otherwise, the recruitment window could be missed. Since making the adaptation means narrowing of the eligibility criteria, this naturally translates to a smaller potential pool of an eligible population, so it can become more difficult to recruit eligible patients, especially if the expected prevalence of the biomarker is low. It is often the case that prevalence of the biomarker is uncertain, so it can be difficult to budget for screening failures or number of biospecimen collections and laboratory tests that can quickly add up in trial cost. Generalisability is also another potential issue for adaptive enrichment designs, especially if the trial ends up making a false enrichment decision. This could mean that potentially effective treatment could be withheld from a larger group of patients who would actually benefit from the treatment.

Seamless Design

Within a traditional clinical drug development program, clinical trials are conducted separately from phase I to phase III designs [74]. The findings from the early phase are used primarily to decide whether further clinical evaluation is warranted. Even if the primary goal of the earlier phase is convincingly met, the clinical drug development program would often 'pause' between phases. Seamless designs are a type of adaptive trial design that allows for immediate continuation from one phase to the subsequent phase [5, 75]. This is useful to shorten the overall time within a clinical drug development program.

As phases IIB and III are similar in their clinical settings, seamless designs are commonly used to seamlessly combine phase II and phase III trials (seamless phase IIB/III) [75, 76]. A seamless phase IIB/III RCT can be feasible even with significant changes to the design across phases, but it does require overlap in some essential components. For example, if a phase IIB trial component examines the tolerability of multiple doses, the successful doses can seamlessly continue onto a phase III portion.

There are two types of seamless designs: (1) operationally seamless, and (2) inferentially seamless [5]. An operationally seamless phase IIB/III design eliminates time between the two phases, but analyses during the phase III portion would not include the data collected from the earlier phase [5]. An inferentially seamless phase IIB/III design, on the other hand, uses data from both phases for analysis [5]. In seamless designs, other types of adaptive trial designs are often commonly used. For instance, there have been seamless phase IIB/III trials with sequential designs that are often used in the phase IIB portion [34, 35, 77, 78].

Seamless designs have the capacity to reduce the time required to complete a clinical drug development program [75]. However, seamless designs require that early data can be rapidly analysed and interpreted to inform decisions about seamless transition into the subsequent phase [75]. Seamless designs also pose challenges in trial administration and infrastructure, as they are often larger than when conducting each trial phase separately [76]. Combining data in an inferentially connected seamless design may require more complex analyses to adjust for patient drift across the combined phases [76]

Conclusion

In this chapter, we have discussed common types of adaptive trial designs and how they use accumulating interim data for pre-specification adaptations. For sequential designs, it is important to pre-specify and to be transparent about the interim analysis plan. This would entail what endpoint and statistical methods will be used, stopping criteria, and when the first interim analysis will occur (burn-in period), and generally how many or how frequently analyses will be conducted. The stopping criteria should be specific and transparent on whether the early stopping for either superiority or futility will be made, or if early stopping for both will be allowed. These transparency considerations, of course, apply to other types of adaptive trial designs as well. In comparison to conventional designs, adaptive trial designs offer more flexibility, but it is important to recognise there is no such thing as free lunch [7]. Trade-offs for the option of flexibility should be carefully considered in advance.

References

1. Dimairo M, Pallmann P, Wason J, et al. The Adaptive designs CONSORT Extension (ACE) statement: a checklist with explanation and elaboration guideline for reporting randomised trials that use an adaptive design. *BMJ.* 2020;**369**:m115.

2. Dimairo M, Pallmann P, Wason J, et al. The Adaptive designs CONSORT Extension (ACE) statement: a checklist with explanation and elaboration guideline for reporting randomised trials that use an adaptive design. *Trials.* 2020;**21**(1):528.

3. Thorlund K, Haggstrom J, Park JJ, Mills EJ. Key design considerations for adaptive clinical trials: a primer for clinicians. *BMJ.* 2018;**360**:k698.

4. Park JJ, Thorlund K, Mills EJ. Critical concepts in adaptive clinical trials. *Clin Epidemiol.* 2018;**10**:343–51.

5. Bhatt DL, Mehta C. Adaptive designs for clinical trials. *N Engl J Med.* 2016;**375** (1):65–74.

6. Pocock SJ. Group sequential methods in the design and analysis of clinical trials. *Biometrika.* 1977;**64**(2):191–9.

7. Bauer P, Bretz F, Dragalin V, Konig F, Wassmer G. Twenty-five years of confirmatory adaptive designs:

opportunities and pitfalls. *Stat Med.* 2016;**35**(3):325–47.

8. Jennison C, Turnbull BW. *Group Sequential Methods with Applications to Clinical Trials.* Chapman and Hall/CRC; 1999.

9. Freidlin B, Korn EL. A comment on futility monitoring. *Control Clin Trials.* 2002;**23** (4):355–66.

10. Saville BR, Connor JT, Ayers GD, Alvarez J. The utility of Bayesian predictive probabilities for interim monitoring of clinical trials. *Clin Trials.* 2014;**11**(4):485–93.

11. Harari O, Hsu G, Dron L, et al. Utilizing Bayesian predictive power in clinical trial design. *Pharm Stat.* 2020.

12. DeMets DL, Pocock SJ, Julian DG. The agonising negative trend in monitoring of clinical trials. *Lancet.* 1999;**354** (9194):1983–8.

13. Ioannidis JP, Evans SJ, Gotzsche PC, et al. Better reporting of harms in randomized trials: an extension of the CONSORT statement. *Ann Intern Med.* 2004;**141** (10):781–8.

14. Pocock SJ. When to stop a clinical trial. *BMJ.* 1992;**305**(6847):235.

15. Armitage P. Sequential medical trials: some comments on FJ Anscombe's paper. *JASA.* 1963;**58**(302):384–7.

16. Armitage P. *Sequential Medical Trials*. Wiley & Sons; 1975.

17. Fleming TR, Harrington DP, O'Brien PC. Designs for group sequential tests. *Control Clin Trials*. 1984;**5**(4):348–61.

18. Pallmann P, Bedding AW, Choodari-Oskooei B, et al. Adaptive designs in clinical trials: why use them, and how to run and report them. *BMC Med*. 2018;**16**(1):29.

19. Berry DA. Bayesian clinical trials. *Nat Rev Drug Discov*. 2006;**5**(1):27–36.

20. Kunzmann K, Grayling MJ, Lee KM, et al. Conditional power and friends: the why and how of (un) planned, unblinded sample size recalculations in confirmatory trials. *Stat Med*. 2022;**41**(5):877–90.

21. Greenland S, Senn SJ, Rothman KJ, et al. Statistical tests, P values, confidence intervals, and power: a guide to misinterpretations. *Eur J Epidemiol*. 2016;**31**(4):337–50.

22. Gordon Lan K, Reboussin DM, DeMets DL. Information and information fractions for design and sequential monitoring of clinical trials. *Commun Stat*. 1994;**23**(2):403–20.

23. O'Brien PC, Fleming TR. A multiple testing procedure for clinical trials. *Biometrics*. 1979;**35**(3):549–56.

24. Haybittle J. Repeated assessment of results in clinical trials of cancer treatment. *Brit J Radiol*. 1971;**44**(526):793–7.

25. Peto R, Pike M, Armitage P, et al. Design and analysis of randomized clinical trials requiring prolonged observation of each patient. I. Introduction and design. *BJC*. 1976;**34**(6):585–612.

26. DeMets DL, Lan KG. Interim analysis: the alpha spending function approach. *Stat Med*. 1994;**13**(13-14):1341–52.

27. Meurer WJ, Tolles J. Interim analyses during group sequential clinical trials. *JAMA*. 2021;**326**(15):1524–5.

28. Lan GK, DeMets DL. Discrete sequential boundaries for clinical trials. *Biometrika*. 1983;**70**(3):659–63.

29. Kim K, DeMets DL. Design and analysis of group sequential tests based on the type I error spending rate function. *Biometrika*. 1987;**74**(1):149–54.

30. Davis BR, Hardy RJ. Data monitoring in clinical trials: the case for stochastic curtailment. *J Clin Epidemiol*. 1994;**47**(9):1033–42.

31. Lakens D, Pahlke F, Wassmer G. Group sequential designs: a tutorial. *PsyArXiv Preprints*. 2021.

32. Green PJ, Łatuszyński K, Pereyra M, Robert CP. Bayesian computation: a summary of the current state, and samples backwards and forwards. *Stat Comput*. 2015;**25**(4):835–62.

33. Spiegelhalter DJ, Freedman LS, Blackburn PR. Monitoring clinical trials: conditional or predictive power? *Control Clin Trials*. 1986;**7**(1):8–17.

34. Park JW, Liu MC, Yee D, et al. Adaptive randomization of neratinib in early breast cancer. *N Engl J Med*. 2016;**375**(1):11–22.

35. Rugo HS, Olopade OI, DeMichele A, et al. Adaptive randomization of veliparib-carboplatin treatment in breast cancer. *N Engl J Med*. 2016;**375**(1):23–34.

36. Viele K, McGlothlin A, Broglio K. Interpretation of clinical trials that stopped early. *JAMA*. 2016;**315**(15):1646–7.

37. Goodman SN. *Stopping at Nothing? Some Dilemmas of Data Monitoring in Clinical Trials*, pp. 882–7. American College of Physicians; 2007.

38. Florey CD. Sample size for beginners. *BMJ*. 1993;**306**(6886):1181–4.

39. Bauer P, Koenig F. The reassessment of trial perspectives from interim data – a critical view. *Stat Med*. 2006;**25**(1):23–36.

40. Posch M, Klinglmueller F, Konig F, Miller F. Estimation after blinded sample size reassessment. *Stat Methods Med Res*. 2018;**27**(6):1830–46.

41. Brannath W, Mehta CR, Posch M. Exact confidence bounds following adaptive group sequential tests. *Biometrics*. 2009;**65**(2):539–46.

42. Kieser M, Friede T. Simple procedures for blinded sample size adjustment that do not

affect the type I error rate. *Stat Med.* 2003;**22**(23):3571–81.

43. Lin J, Lin L-A, Sankoh S. A general overview of adaptive randomization design for clinical trials. *J Biom Biostat.* 2016;**7**(2):294.

44. Lin Y, Zhu M, Su Z. The pursuit of balance: an overview of covariate-adaptive randomization techniques in clinical trials. *Contemp Clin Trials.* 2015;**45**(Pt A):21–5.

45. Atkinson AC, Biswas A. *Randomised Response-Adaptive Designs in Clinical Trials.* CRC Press; 2013.

46. Taves DR. Minimization: a new method of assigning patients to treatment and control groups. *Clin Pharmacol Ther.* 1974;**15**(5):443–53.

47. Pocock SJ, Simon R. Sequential treatment assignment with balancing for prognostic factors in the controlled clinical trial. *Biometrics.* 1975;**31**(1):103–15.

48. Altman DG, Bland JM. Treatment allocation by minimisation. *BMJ.* 2005;**330**(7495):843.

49. Zajicek J, Ball S, Wright D, et al. Effect of dronabinol on progression in progressive multiple sclerosis (CUPID): a randomised, placebo-controlled trial. *Lancet Neurol.* 2013;**12**(9):857–65.

50. Treasure T, MacRae KD. Minimisation: the platinum standard for trials? Randomisation doesn't guarantee similarity of groups; minimisation does. *BMJ.* 1998;**317**(7155):362–3.

51. Rosenberger WF, Lachin JM. *Randomization in Clinical Trials: Theory and Practice.* Wiley & Sons; 2015.

52. Saghaei M. An overview of randomization and minimization programs for randomized clinical trials. *J Med Signals Sens.* 2011;**1**(1):55–61.

53. Angus DC. Optimizing the trade-off between learning and doing in a pandemic. *JAMA.* 2020;**323**(19):1895–6.

54. Creel AH, Losina E, Mandl LA, et al. An assessment of willingness to participate in a randomized trial of arthroscopic knee surgery in patients with osteoarthritis. *Contemp Clin Trials.* 2005;**26**(2):169–78.

55. Proschan M, Evans S. Resist the temptation of response-adaptive randomization. *Clin Infect Dis.* 2020;**71**(11):3002–4.

56. Viele K, Broglio K, McGlothlin A, Saville BR. Comparison of methods for control allocation in multiple arm studies using response adaptive randomization. *Clin Trials.* 2020;**17**(1):52–60.

57. Thall P, Fox P, Wathen J. Statistical controversies in clinical research: scientific and ethical problems with adaptive randomization in comparative clinical trials. *Ann Oncol.* 2015;**26**(8):1621–8.

58. Wathen JK, Thall PF. A simulation study of outcome adaptive randomization in multi-arm clinical trials. *Clin Trials.* 2017;**14**(5):432–40.

59. London AJ. Learning health systems, clinical equipoise and the ethics of response adaptive randomisation. *J Med Ethics.* 2018;**44**(6):409–15.

60. Meurer WJ, Lewis RJ, Berry DA. Adaptive clinical trials: a partial remedy for the therapeutic misconception? *JAMA.* 2012;**307**(22):2377–8.

61. Tehranisa JS, Meurer WJ. Can response-adaptive randomization increase participation in acute stroke trials? *Stroke.* 2014;**45**(7):2131–3.

62. Thompson WR. On the likelihood that one unknown probability exceeds another in view of the evidence of two samples. *Biometrika.* 1933;**25**(3-4):285–94.

63. Juszczak E, Altman DG, Hopewell S, Schulz K. Reporting of multi-arm parallel-group randomized trials: extension of the consort 2010 statement. *JAMA.* 2019;**321**(16):1610–20.

64. Koenig F, Brannath W, Bretz F, Posch M. Adaptive Dunnett tests for treatment selection. *Stat Med.* 2008;**27**(10):1612–25.

65. Zhao W, Durkalski V. Managing competing demands in the implementation of response-adaptive randomization in a large multicenter phase III acute stroke trial. *Stat Med* 2014;**33**(23):4043–52.

66. Treweek S, Pitkethly M, Cook J, et al. Strategies to improve recruitment to randomised trials. *Cochrane Database Syst Rev.* 2018;**2**:MR000013.

67. Hodson R. Precision oncology. *Nature.* 2020;**585**(7826):S1.

68. Simon N, Simon R. Adaptive enrichment designs for clinical trials. *Biostatistics.* 2013;**14**(4):613–25.

69. Antoniou M, Jorgensen AL, Kolamunnage-Dona R. Biomarker-guided adaptive trial designs in phase II and phase III: a methodological review. *PLoS One.* 2016;**11**(2):e0149803.

70. Antoniou M, Kolamunnage-Dona R, Jorgensen AL. Biomarker-guided non-adaptive trial designs in phase II and phase III: a methodological review. *J Pers Med.* 2017;**7**(1).

71. Mehta CR, Gao P. Population enrichment designs: case study of a large multinational trial. *J Biopharm Stat.* 2011;**21**(4):831–45.

72. Nogueira RG, Jadhav AP, Haussen DC, et al. Thrombectomy 6 to 24 hours after stroke with a mismatch between deficit and infarct. *N Engl J Med.* 2018;**378**(1):11–21.

73. Antoniou M, Kolamunnage-Dona R, Wason J, et al. Biomarker-guided trials: Challenges in practice. *Contemp Clin Trials Commun.* 2019;**16**:100493.

74. Grudzinskas C. Design of clinical development programs. In Atkinson AJ, Abernethy DR, Daniels CE, Dedrick RL, Markey SP, editors. *Principles of Clinical Pharmacology*, 2nd ed., pp. 501–17. Academic Press; 2007.

75. Cuffe RL, Lawrence D, Stone A, Vandemeulebroecke M. When is a seamless study desirable? Case studies from different pharmaceutical sponsors. *Pharmaceutical statistics.* 2014;**13**(4):229–37.

76. Hobbs BP, Barata PC, Kanjanapan Y, et al. Seamless designs: current practice and considerations for early-phase drug development in oncology. *J Natl Cancer Inst.* 2019;**111**(2):118–28.

77. Sydes MR, Parmar MK, Mason MD, et al. Flexible trial design in practice – stopping arms for lack-of-benefit and adding research arms mid-trial in STAMPEDE: a multi-arm multi-stage randomized controlled trial. *Trials.* 2012;**13**:168.

78. Barker AD, Sigman CC, Kelloff GJ, et al. I-SPY 2: an adaptive breast cancer trial design in the setting of neoadjuvant chemotherapy. *Clin Pharmacol Ther.* 2009;**86**(1):97–100.

Clinical Trial Simulations

Jay J. H. Park, Edward Mills, and J. Kyle Wathen

Key Points of This Chapter
In this chapter, we discuss clinical trial simulations from the concept of simulation-guided trial designs with examples. The key points of this chapter are: • Clinical trial simulation is required to explore, compare, and characterise operating characteristics and statistical properties of adaptive and other innovative trials with complex designs. • Clinical trial simulation is an important tool that allows for comparison of different design choices during the planning stage to enhance the quality and feasibility of the trial. While simulations are most frequently used in adaptive and other complex trial designs, they can be applied to fixed trial designs. • There are both commercial and non-commercial clinical trial simulation software programs available. Each software program allows simulations of specific adaptive trial designs that have been pre-developed. Non-commercial simulation software programs are becoming increasingly available.

Introduction

Simulation in statistics generally refers to repeated analyses of randomly generated datasets with known properties. Datasets are repeatedly drawn under assumptions made on the data-generating mechanism and design specifications. As an illustrative example of simulations, let us consider a simple coin flip. A single coin flip is an example of an experiment with a binary outcome, since in a two-sided coin flip, there are two possible outcomes: heads (H) and tails (T). Each outcome has a fixed and equal probability of 1/2 (50%). It is likely the reader may have seen similar examples of a coin toss being used to illustrate the concept of binomial distribution in their Statistics course.

Regardless, let us a consider a question: 'Given a fair coin, what is the probability of getting 5 heads out of 10 flips?' If one manually flipped the coin 10 times, they might get 3 heads and 7 tails. If they flipped the coin 10 more this, they would likely get a different outcome and we ought to be sceptical in a claim such as the probability of getting 5 heads is 0. Instead, we can intuitively say this happened just by random chance and 5 heads out of 10 flips is most likely. Given the law of large numbers, we need to repeat the 10 coin tosses many times (e.g., 1,000) to obtain a reliable estimate of the probability of getting 5 heads out of 10 flips. Instead of manually tossing the coins and recording the results many times, we can just use a computer program, such as R, to estimate the probability of 5 heads based on

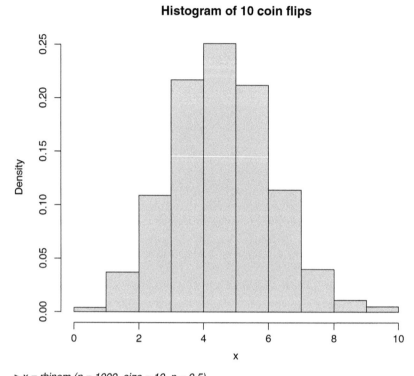

```
> x = rbinom (n = 1000, size = 10, p = 0.5)

> hist(x, probability = TRUE, main = "Histogram of 10 coin flips")
```

Figure 5.1 Simulated probability of heads in 10 coin flips.

a few simple lines of codes. Here in Figure 5.1, we can see a histogram of 10 coin flips with a fair 2-sided coin that were repeated 1,000 times. Instead of manually tossing the coins, we can use simulations to repeat the procedure of 'flipping' the coin 10 times and record the number of heads many times to answer the question of interest.

When statisticians discuss clinical trial simulation, they usually mean Monte Carlo simulation studies [1]. Monte Carlo simulation is a method of estimating the value of unknown quantity by repeatedly taking a random sample. Simulating a clinical trial requires one to specify all trial design details, such as sample size, analysis method(s), interim analysis plan, and decision rules. It also requires one to specify all simulation scenarios that contain information such as true parameter values for patient simulation, patient recruitment rates, and patient drop out models (more details on clinical trial simulation are provided in the next section). Patient data are generated accordingly, then the statistical analysis is applied to the data. Simulation uses computer algorithm to repeat the process many times, with the results of each trial being stored. This repeated random sampling process allows us to examine how the statistical procedure performs at recovering, or estimating, the 'known' true parameter values that we have specified for the simulation. The general step of simulation with the coin toss example is illustrated in Table 5.1.

Table 5.1 General overview of simulations
The general steps of simulations with the detailed breakdown of the coin-toss simulation are provided in this table.

General steps	Applied to the coin toss example
Choose data-generating mechanism	Discrete events (heads or tails) generated from a binomial distribution
Specify numerical values for:	
• Simulation parameters	Probability of heads = 0.50
• Sample size	10 tosses of the coin
• Analysis/test statistic	Number of heads out of the 10 tosses
Choose number of replications	1,000 times
For each replication:	
A. Generate data according to the model and parameters	Generate 10 random coin tosses
B. Run analysis	Count the number of heads out of 10 tosses
C. Keep track of the performance	Keep track of B and repeat 1,000 times
Display the results	See Figure 5.1

The use of simulation has a wide range of possible utility for clinical trials and other areas in medical research. Simulation studies allow us to assess the performance of statistical methods, design options, and explore their properties under varying conditions and parameters [2, 3]. Most statistical methods are developed under specific assumptions; however, since these assumptions cannot be validated in a real-life setting, it is much more practical to use computer simulations to understand how departures from the assumptions impact the clinical trial and results. We often rely on simulations to evaluate appropriateness and accuracy of statistical methods under conditions that we can specify [2]. Simulation studies comparing the performance of different competing trial designs can allow one to determine which method is most appropriate in a particular setting and access potential problems with the trial design. Therefore, the utility of simulation studies in a clinical trial design process has become very important. In this chapter, we discuss important concepts and terminologies of clinical trial simulation and the principles of simulation-guided trial design. We discuss the general overview of simulation procedures, the importance of carefully thinking about what scenarios need to be simulated, the role and importance of simulation reports, and lastly available simulation software that readers can use.

Clinical Trial Simulation

Terminology

- **Operating characteristics** (synonym: performance metrics) are descriptions of how a design performs under various scenarios. Common examples of operating characteristics include but are not limited to type I error rate, power, average sample size, average trial duration, probability of success.
- **Scenario** refers to a list of values specifying the 'true' underlying parameters, such as true response rates, recruitment rate, and/or patient drop-out rates. One may think of

a scenario as a complete list of the assumed values for all the parameters that one does not know or does not have the ability to control in a clinical trial.

- **Simulation** refers to repeated analyses of randomly generated datasets drawn under specific assumptions in a scenario and trial design. It involves a process of generating random patient outcomes from 'known' properties using computers software (data-generating mechanism) and applying the specific trial design that includes specific statistical analysis (statistical model).
- **Simulation report** (synonym: adaptive trial design report) refers to a written document that provides the explanation, details, and justification of the simulation study. As a supporting document to the main trial protocol, a simulation report contains methodological details and summary of findings from the simulations conducted. This document is helpful in understanding the scenarios where the trial design will perform well and also how to explain any limitations of the design and/or simulations study.
- **Trial design** refers to the details about how the trial is conducted, including sample size, interim analysis plan, analysis details, decision rule, and any details about features that may be adapted or changed during the trial.
- **Virtual trial** refers to the clinical trial being simulated *in silico*. The virtual trial enrols virtual patients via simulation in order to understand how the trial may perform and make decisions when the clinical trial is conducted.

Overview of Clinical Trial Simulation

The use of clinical trial simulation has become more common over the years. With adaptive trial designs becoming a cornerstone of pharmaceutical research and development (R&D), the uptake of clinical trial simulation has increased. For adaptive and other complex innovative trials, the regulatory authorities often mandate use of clinical trial simulation because the operating characteristics and statistical properties of adaptive decisions cannot be derived analytically without simulations [4–6]. In addition, there has been increasing awareness of how clinical trial simulation can be used as an effective clinical development strategy [4, 7]. Clinical trial simulation provides a formal analytical framework in which one can gain an understanding of how a given trial will perform under different scenarios to better characterise the uncertainties around their benefits and risks. Following the principle of simulation-guided trial design [8], multiple design options can be compared in the planning stage in terms of their relative risks and benefits to carefully choose an efficient trial design that is most likely to address the question(s) the trial is designed to answer.

The goal of clinical trial simulation is to make virtual trial design match as closely as possible how the trial will be conducted. In clinical trial simulation, the virtual trial is simulated repeatedly by enrolling computer-generated patients under a scenario defined by specific parameters and conditions, such as true response and recruitment rates, to obtain average behaviour or operating characteristics of the trial design. The common operating characteristics of interest include false-positive error rate, statistical power, average sample size, and trial duration. The general steps of simulation for an adaptive clinical trial would involve:

- Step 1: Simulate the arrival time of the next patient.
- Step 2: Check the stopping rules to see if the trial should be stopped.
- Step 3: If the trial is not stopped, enrol more patients into the next interim analysis.

- Step 4: Simulate the patient outcome as a function of the treatment; this also includes the time the outcome is observed.
- Step 5: Repeat steps 1–4.

Principles of Simulation-Guided Trial Design

The simulation-guided trial design process aims to integrate relevant information available during the design stage and critically assess how deviations from the assumptions will impact the operating characteristics in an analytical manner [9, 10]. Regardless of whether the final chosen design is adaptive or not, the simulation-guided design process that considers multiple design candidates should be a routine practice [7]. No trial designs should be used by default. We remain enthusiastic about adaptive trials; however, it cannot be said that they should be used for all clinical questions. There are many instances where adaptive trial designs lead to important efficiency gains over fixed trial designs, but there are instances in which adaptive trial designs are not useful [11]. Every clinical question deserves a thorough investigation and consideration of the pros and cons when selecting design options, and there should be no default design choice. An efficient trial design for one research question can be inefficient for another. Trial planning practices should include considerations of multiple designs using clinical trial simulations to weigh the pros and cons of each design to inform an efficient trial design for the given clinical question in conjunction with other factors.

For the right question, adaptive trial designs have the potential to reduce resource requirements, decrease time to completion, reduce the number of patients exposed to inferior interventions, and improve the likelihood of success of the clinical trial. With any adaptation, one should judiciously and rigorously assert that the likelihood of scientific and ethical gains outweighs the risk associated with such an adaptation. It is often helpful to anticipate particular study outcomes that could lead to failure so as to ask what planning decisions one might later regret. This concept is called 'anticipated regret'. For example, if a study just barely missed its objective but still had a clinically important effect and in retrospect would have likely succeeded if the sample size had been slightly larger, that might suggest that one should have planned for an adaptive sample size design in which the sample size could be reassessed partway through the study. The ability to anticipate what one might regret and then planning areas of adaptive trial designs around these areas can be effective in increasing the likelihood of study success. Adaptive designs that rely on anticipated regret can decrease the uncertainty in studies and make them much more predictable. Such planning can be thought of as insurance against possible threats to the success of the study. Preferably using clinical trial simulations, one can calculate the costs associated with such insurance by comparing an adaptive design to a fixed sample design.

Example of Clinical Trial Simulation

For examples of ready-made clinical trial simulations, we refer the reader to three examples of clinical trial simulations that can be found in this GitHub repository: https://github.com/kwathen/IntroBayesianSimulation. The goal of this repository is to focus on how to develop the necessary R code to simulate a Bayesian response adaptive randomisation, where randomisation probabilities are altered prior to each patient enrolling, and for the possibility of early stopping for superiority or futility. The examples provided in the repository focus on the necessary steps and skills required to develop a custom simulation package. Through a series of three examples, where each example builds on the previous, the R code necessary for simulation of the desired adaptive design is developed in a stepwise fashion. As such, each example in this repository is a self-contained R project to simulate a design.

Simulation-Guided Design Planning Case Study

In the clinical design process, simulations are highly iterative, with teams typically performing many rounds of simulations as the design priorities and goals evolve. In this section, we focus on going beyond the usual operating characteristics and average behaviour to understand more about trade-offs between different designs, and how the simulations can help the team understand which design option(s) are most likely to help achieve a desired outcome. This section does not aim to recommend one design choice as superior but rather utilises a Bayesian adaptive approach to illustrate various metrics that the team reviews.

Design and Scenario Assumptions

In the remainder of this section, we utilise the 'Example3' folder in the GitHub repository to demonstrate the principle of simulation-guided design. We considered three design options and three scenarios as outlined in Table 5.2. All three designs compare the response rate on the Standard-of-Care and Experimental arms enrolling a maximum sample size of 200 patients with interim analyses being conducted every 10 patients after a minimum sample size (burn-in) of 30 patients. In other words, the accrual of the trial may stop after 30 (minimum), 40, 50, 60, 70, 80, 90, 100, 110, 120, 130, 140, 150, 160, 170, 180, 190, or 200 (maximum) subjects.

With higher response rate indicating more favourable clinical outcome, we assume there is a 1-month delay between treatment and evaluation of the patient's binary response. To simulate the virtual trials, we assume, on average, that 10 patients per month are enrolled

Table 5.2 Overview of trial designs and scenarios

No.	Trial designs	Scenarios
1	*Equal randomisation* -1:1 allocation to E and S	*Equal treatment effect/response rate (Null)* - pS = 0.3 and pE = 0.3
2	*RAR with no minimum/maximum allocation* - At interim analysis, adapt the allocation probability for E to probability that E has higher response rate than S (p_E) - Allocation of S would be $1 - p_E$	*10% higher response rate in E* - pS = 0.3 and pE = 0.4
3	*RAR with minimum/maximum allocation* - Same as Design 2 with 10% minimum and 90% maximal allocation probabilities, to ensure that the allocation does not get 'stuck' on one study arm	*20% higher response rate in E* - pS = 0.3 and pE = 0.5

E = experimental arm, S = standard-of-care arm; RAR = response adaptive randomisation; pS = Response rate of S; pE = Response rate of E where enrolment times are simulated from a Poisson process. We denote the response rate on the Standard-of-Care by pS and the Experimental by pE. We assume, a priori, pS~Beta(0.2, 0.8) and pE~Beta(0.2, 0.8), which is equivalent to a prior sample size of 1 patient with a response rate of 20% and reflects equipoise.

All three designs allow for early stopping based on superiority, if the response rate of the Experimental is greater than the Standard-of-Care, or futility if it is very unlikely that the Experimental provides a benefit over the Standard-of-Care. The thresholds for superiority and futility are 0.995% and 0.005, respectively. The numerical value of 0.995 was selected to control the expected type I error rate below 3.3% based on the null hypothesis scenario (Scenario 1) that assumed no treatment effects. The percentage of virtual trials that ended up selecting the Experimental as being superior at the end of the trial of the null hypothesis scenario indicates our expected type I error rate for each trial design. For the other scenarios that the Experimental would be more effective (indicated by the higher response rate), the percentage of virtual trials that ended up the Experimental arm indicates our expected statistical power.

The three designs differ by their allocation strategies. The first design, Design 1, uses an equal allocation design. The Designs 2 and 3 use response adaptive randomisation designs, where the allocation ratio for the Experimental arm is adjusted based on the probability that the Experimental arm has a higher response rate than the Standard-of-Care arm at each interim analysis. At the interim, we compute the posterior probability of superiority for the Experimental, $\text{Prob}(pE > pS \mid \text{data})$, to update the allocation ratio for Designs 2 and 3. Since there are only two arms, the allocation ratio for the Standard-of-Care arm can be calculated by subtracting the superiority of Experimental from 1. The difference between Design 2 and Design 3 is the specification of the minimum and maximum allocation ratios in Design 3. We used a minimum allocation ratio of 10% and a maximum allocation ratio of 90% to ensure that the allocation does not get 'stuck' to one study arm.

Simulation Results

To compare the design options, 10,000 virtual trials were simulated for each scenario. The operating characteristics are provided in Table 5.3 for each design and scenario. As indicated by the percentage of virtual trials where the Experimental arm was determined to be superior to the Standard-of-Care (% of superiority for Exp), the expected type I error rate and expected power can be seen under the null effect and alternative effects scenarios. All three designs have similar expected type I error rates ranging from 0.030 to 0.032. The expected power is generally low across all designs in Scenario 2, where only 10% higher response rate is assumed for the Experimental arm. The Design 2 without no minimum or maximum allocation had the lowest power at 0.15; where the Design 1 with fixed allocation design had the highest power at 0.24. In Scenario 3, where 20% higher response rate is assumed for the Experimental arm in comparison to the Standard-of-Care, the power for Design 1 is 0.72 but lower for the RAR designs (0.43 and 0.56). This is not surprising since in two-arm clinical trial setting, adopting an equal allocation will have the highest power compared to unequal allocation (e.g., 2:1 allocation). By having the minimum and maximum allocation ratios in Design 3, we can see there is marginal gain in statistical power over Design 2, where there is no minimum/maximum allocation ratio specified.

The percentage of virtual trials that stopped prior to the maximum sample size (% of early stopping), average sample size (2.5%, 97.5%), and average trial duration (in months) are also shown in Table 5.3. They are useful operating characteristics for operational planning and financial considerations. We can see that the response adaptive randomisation designs, on average, are producing equal sample size designs under the null effect scenario, and unequal allocation designs for the Scenarios 2 and 3 as intended, where the Experimental arm is assumed to be superior to the Standard-of-Care arm. However, it is critical that we go beyond these average operating characteristics that are usually reported to truly gain a deeper understanding of the potential risks of each design.

It is possible in response adaptive randomisation to have the opposite unintended effect where more patients end up being assigned to the inferior treatment arm [12]. However, this is not usually apparent and obvious upon examination of the usual operating characteristics, such as average sample size. For instance, we provide the percentage of trials where at least more than 20 patients ended up being assigned to the Standard-of-Care arm versus the Experimental arm. In a two-arm trial size of 200 patients, an imbalance of 20 patients represents a significant difference that is beyond random chance, so this was used for our simulation. The proportion of trials where at least 20 patients ended up being allocated to the Standard-of-Care over the Experimental arm (P20) is shown in the last column of Table 5.3. In the null effect scenario, P20 is 0.07. We did not specify the use of permuted block randomisation that could guarantee exactly 100 patients being allocated to each arm, so there is small chance of imbalance even for the Design 1. Even though our estimated sample size, on average, is generally equal, under the null effect scenario, the estimated P20 for both of the response adaptive randomisation designs is more drastic. They each showed 42% of the simulated virtual trials of response adaptive randomisation designs resulted in at least 20 patients being allocated to the Standard-of-Care arm. This is likely not what we want when considering response adaptive randomisation that is motivated by the desire to assign more patients to the 'better' treatment.

Examination of Single Virtual Trials

We usually repeat simulations many times to adhere to the law of large numbers and to avoid Monte Carlo errors. However, it is important to note that a trial in reality will be conducted only once. It is therefore critical to look at examples of single virtual trials to understand how the trial may progress to illuminate many potential issues that may arise. The specific details of what needs to be looked at depends on the nature of the trial designs and should be tailored to investigate any of the planned adaptations.

For Scenario 1 (null effect), the randomisation probability of the Experimental arm (E) over the total sample size from 0 to 200 from three virtual trials is plotted in Figure 5.2. For Scenario 2 (10% higher response rate in the Experimental arm), the same plots are provided for six virtual trials but separated into two plots, Figure 5.3 and Figure 5.4. For this discussion, we are not showing examples of virtual trials for Scenario 3, but readers can refer to the GitHub repository to examine the virtual trials for themselves. In each figure, all designs had the same burn-in of 30 patients at equal randomisation and same patient outcomes, so that after the initial set of patients everything was as similar as possible and the differences are only due to the RAR after that point.

In Figure 5.2, which is the null case, the three virtual trials for Design 2 (row 2) show that there is a non-trivial chance that the RAR will favour one treatment even when there is no difference. For example, for Design 2, Virtual Trial 3, the randomisation favoured S and assigned considerably more patients to the Standard-of-Care than the Experimental arm,

Table 5.3 Summary of simulation results

The operating characteristics to compare Designs 1–3 for the three different scenarios. The '% of superiority for Exp' column provides the percentage of virtual trials that deemed the Experimental arm to be superior (0.995) over the Standard-of-Care arm. The '% of early stopping' column provides the percentage of virtual trials that ended early before 200 patients. The 'P20' column provides the percentage of virtual trials that enrolled at least 20 more patients on the SOC arm over the Exp arm.

Design	% of superiority for Exp	% of early stopping	Average sample size (2.5%, 97.5%)			Average trial duration (months)	P20
			Exp	SOC	Total		
Scenario 1: Null effect							
1: Fixed	0.032	0.062	96 (27,114)	97 (27,113)	193 (49,200)	20	0.07
2: RAR no min/max	0.030	0.058	96 (18,177)	96 (18,178)	193 (49,200)	20	0.42
3: RAR with min/max	0.033	0.063	95 (22,167)	97 (23,168)	192 (49,200)	20	0.42
Scenario 2: 10% higher response rate in experimental arm							
1: Fixed	0.24	0.23	89 (21,113)	90 (21,114)	179 (39,200)	19	0.06
2: RAR no min/max	0.15	0.15	128 (24,182)	56 (14,155)	183 (39,200)	19	0.10
3: RAR with min/max	0.19	0.18	124 (26,171)	58 (16,149)	182 (39,200)	19	0.10
Scenario 3: 20% higher response rate in experimental arm							
1: Fixed	0.72	0.69	68 (18,110)	68 (18,110)	136 (39,200)	14	0.04
2: RAR no min/max	0.43	0.42	123 (23,183)	32 (12, 90)	155 (39,200)	16	0.01
3: RAR with min/max	0.56	0.54	111 (22,172)	36 (14,88)	147 (39,200)	15	0.01

Exp = Experimental arm; SOC = Standard-of-care arm

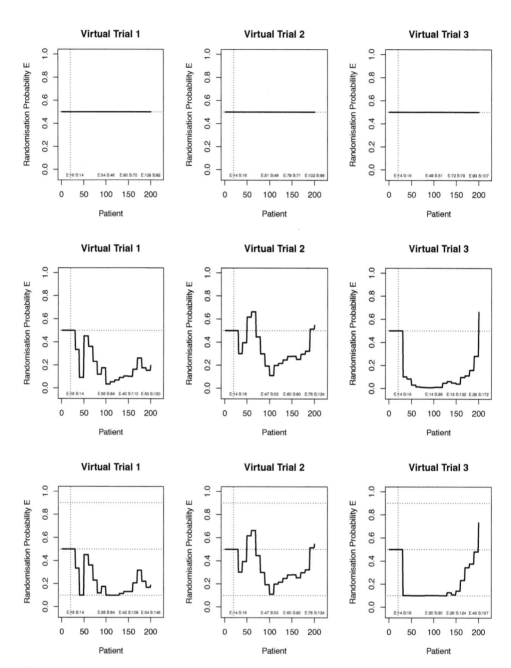

Figure 5.2 Randomisation probabilities of Scenario 1 (null effect): Virtual Trials 1–3.

In this scenario of null effect (Scenario 1), equal response rates were assumed between the Experimental (E) and Standard-of-Care (S).

Numbers displayed at the bottom of each graph are the number of patients on E and S when the initial randomisation of 30 patients completes, 100 patients, 150 patients and 200 patients enrolled. The first row illustrates three virtual trials of Design 1; the second row for Design 2; and the last row for Design 3.

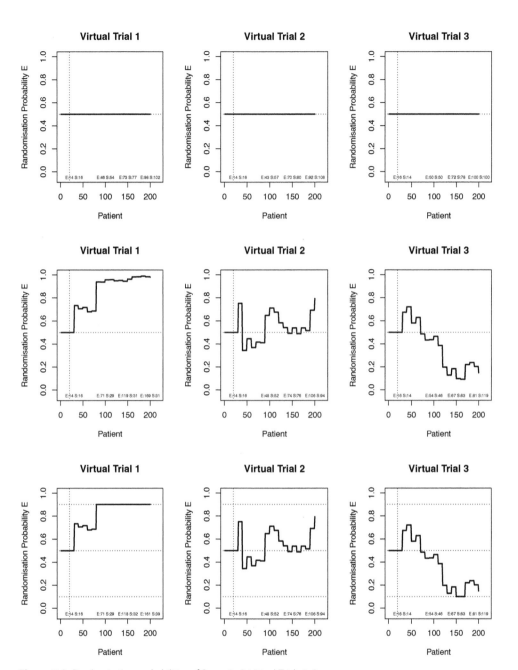

Figure 5.3 Randomisation probabilities of Scenario 2: Virtual Trials 1–3.

In this scenario of alternative effect (Scenario 2), the Experimental (E) arm is assumed to have 10% higher response than the Standard-of-Care (S).

Numbers displayed at the bottom of each graph are the number of patients on E and S when the initial randomisation of 30 patients completes, 100 patients, 150 patients and 200 patients enrolled. The first row illustrates three virtual trials of Design 1; the second row for Design 2; and the last row for Design 3.

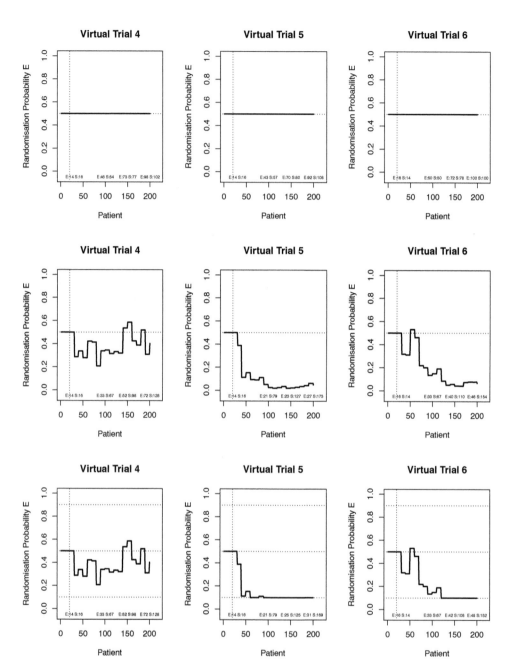

Figure 5.4 Randomisation probabilities of Scenario 2: Virtual Trials 4–6.

In this scenario of alternative effect (Scenario 3), the Experimental (E) arm is assumed to have 20% higher response than the Standard-of-Care (S).

Numbers displayed at the bottom of each graph are the number of patients on E and S when the initial randomisation of 30 patients completes, 100 patients, 150 patients and 200 patients enrolled. The first row illustrates three virtual trials of Design 1; the second row for Design 2; and the last row for Design 3.

172 versus 26, respectively. One of the goals of putting a minimum randomisation in place when using response adaptive randomisation is to help keep the procedure from being 'stuck' in assigning one treatment. For Design 3, Virtual Trial 3, the minimum randomisation probability, shown by the dotted horizontal lines, causes the randomisation to add more patients to the Experimental arm, when compared to Design 2 such that the sample size imbalance is more even, 43 on the Experimental and 157 on Standard-of-Care.

This is not to illustrate by one example that all response adaptive randomisation procedures are flawed, but rather to highlight how the minimum randomisation probability would impact the trial. One must question the clinical development team whether it would be acceptable for the trial to pan out like the Virtual Trial 3. If not, at the design stage changes can be made, such as having a longer burn-in, slowing the adaption, or increasing the minimum randomisation probability. However, it is difficult to draw a broad general conclusion, and these types of detailed trade-offs must be carefully considered to understand the merits of each design option.

In Figure 5.3 and Figure 5.4, six virtual trials that were simulated under Scenario 2 (experimental has 10% higher response rate) are shown. Virtual Trial 1 shows a trial that really benefitted from the response adaptive randomisation and many more patients received the superior treatment, 169 versus 31 for Design 2 and 161 versus 39 for Design 3 (Figure 5.3). The Virtual Trial 2 had almost equal randomisation for all three designs. The Virtual Trial 3 shows an illustration of how response adaptive randomisation, in Design 2 or 3, can imbalance in the wrong direction and assign more patients to the inferior treatment by a large margin in this case, 36 more patients on E for both Design 2 and 3. In Figure 5.4, all three virtual trials (Virtual Trials 4–6) for Designs 2 and 3 ended with considerably more patients on Standard-of-Care than on the Experimental arm. These results show why a metric like P20 in Table 5.3 is important to include, such that the clinical development team can understand the risk of using a response adaptive randomisation procedure. While the response adaptive randomisation is shown to be problematic in this example, for the right research question, it can be beneficial. However, it will be important to consider the trade-offs of such designs using simulations. Instead of selecting a new approach due to its apparent novelty and theoretical benefits, it is critical to understand the trade-offs and carefully consider many design options, since there is no one best design that uniformly applies to all clinical questions.

Simulation Report

Transparency in clinical trial research is an important requirement. To reduce barriers in communication of statistical design aspects of adaptive trial designs and other complex trials, there has been increasing emphasis on adopting a unifying framework for simulation reports [4]. A simulation report, which has been referred to as an adaptive trial design report, is a key document that provides justification of statistical design. For adaptive trial designs, the simulation report is a required document for regulatory and ethics approvals [4]

Under the Drug Information Association Adaptive Design Scientific Working Group (DIA-ADSWG), a group of statisticians with expertise and decades of experience working on adaptive trial designs in 2019 published their recommendations for simulation practices and key elements that should be included in simulation reports [4]. The recommended general contents of a simulation report are illustrated in Table 5.4. In brief, a simulation

Table 5.4 General contents of a simulation report

Sections	Sub-sections
Introduction	• Study objectives • Clinical trial simulation objectives
Simulation input and methods	• Design candidates and their rationale • Interim analyses and decision rules • Data-generating model • Scenarios • Operating characteristics of interest
Simulation results	• Average operating characteristics results
Discussion	• Highlights of the recommended design and relevant results
Conclusion	• Summary of the recommended design
References	• Relevant literature for key design assumptions, etc.

report should include the objectives of the study and clinical trial simulation, simulation inputs and methods, results, and summaries [4]. Since adaptive clinical trials often use more than one specific type of adaptive trial design, it is critical to highlight the differences and their trade-offs in different scenarios that provided justification to the final chosen design. This article by DIA-ADSWG members largely reflect the perspective of clinical trials sponsored by pharmaceutical companies for registrational purposes, but these general simulation practices can be extended outside of pharmaceutical R&D.

Simulation Software

There is commercial and non-commercial software available for clinical trial simulations [13]. Notable commercial simulation software includes EAST®, ADDPLAN®, COMPASS® 2.0, and FACTS. Albeit at cost, commercial software can have important advantages over non-commercial software. Pay-to-use software will offer the convenience of having pre-pared tools that can facilitate the comparison of multiple trial designs in a timely manner. As they are already developed, there is no development time required for the users. Without the need for experience and knowledge of programming languages, the users can utilise the software to simulate multiple candidate design options with inputs of their choice. These commercial tools also often come with support for users as well. While some companies will offer discounts to academics, the cost for licensing can still be prohibitive. Commercial software also often cannot be extended to handle new custom simulations of new trial designs that are not available in the software.

For non-commercial software, it is important to mention the increasing role of R in biostatistics including clinical trial research [14]. R is a free programming language with a growing community of developers, collaborators, testers, and more. Over the years, there have been an increasing number of R packages being developed for clinical trial simulations and statistical analyses [13, 15-17]. The list of notable non-commercial software available in forms of R packages is provided in Table 5.5. They are highlighted here since they provide long-from guide documentation (called vignettes) as tutorials on how to use their

Table 5.5 Notable R packages for clinical trial simulation of adaptive trial designs

Package name – Full name URL
'Rpact' – *Confirmatory Adaptive Clinical Trial Design and Analysis* https://cran.r-project.org/web/packages/rpact/index.html
'MAMS' – *Designing Multi-Arm Multi-Stage Studies* https://cran.r-project.org/web/packages/MAMS/index.html
'Mediana' – *an R package for clinical trial simulations* https://cran.r-project.org/web/packages/Mediana/vignettes/mediana.html
'Multiarm' – *Design of single- and multi-stage multi-arm clinical trials [15]* https://mjgrayling.shinyapps.io/multiarm/ https://github.com/mjg211/multiarm
'adaptr' – *Adaptive Trial Simulator [18]* https://cran.r-project.org/web/packages/adaptr/index.html
'OCTOPUS' – *Optimize Clinical Trials On Platforms Using Simulation Update* https://github.com/kwathen/OCTOPUS
gsDesign https://cran.r-project.org/web/packages/gsDesign/index.html https://keaven.github.io/gsDesign/

This is not a comprehensive list of non-commercial software. A more comprehensive list of software is provided in Meyer et al., 2021 [13] and on the Comprehensive R Archive Network (CRAN), https://cran.r-project.org/web/packages/available_packages_by_name.html.

R packages for simulating common design features and endpoints for the readers. The M. D. Anderson software download site also provides a wide variety of free software for simulating Bayesian designs (https://biostatistics.mdanderson.org/SoftwareDownload/).

The goal of simulation-guided design should explore multiple candidate design options to identify the most efficient design for the clinical question under investigation, so it is important not to change the trial design to match the available design options in the software, whether they are free or commercial. It is often the case that custom simulation design, even if it is a one-off solution, is needed to be developed to address different adaptive elements for a given research question. Since such customisation will require developers with expertise and knowledge of clinical trial designs and programming, as well as time for development, this can be prohibitive. As a general rule of thumb, it is important to identify statisticians with expertise in clinical trial simulations and to engage them early for the planning of your clinical trial.

Conclusion

Clinical trial simulation is a requirement for many adaptive and other innovative trials with complex statistical design to explore, compare, and characterise their operating characteristics and statistical properties. Simulation is an effective tool that can optimise trial planning since it provides a formal analytical framework in which multiple candidate design options can be explored in different scenarios to come up with a final design that is efficient for a given research question. When simulating adaptive designs, the reported results should include metrics to help the clinical development team understand the benefits and risks of each design option, as there is rarely a universally superior design choice.

References

1. Gasparini A, Morris TP, Crowther MJ. INTEREST: INteractive Tool for Exploring REsults from Simulation sTudies. *J Data Sci Stat Vis.* 2021;**1**(4).

2. Burton A, Altman DG, Royston P, Holder RL. The design of simulation studies in medical statistics. *Stat Med.* 2006;**25**(24):4279–92.

3. Boulesteix AL, Groenwold RH, Abrahamowicz M, et al. Introduction to statistical simulations in health research. *BMJ Open.* 2020;**10**(12):e039921.

4. Mayer C, Perevozskaya I, Leonov S, et al. Simulation practices for adaptive trial designs in drug and device development. *Stat Biopharm Res.* 2019;**11**(4):325–35.

5. United States Department of Health and Human Services, Food and Drug Administration. *Adaptive Designs for Clinical Trials of Drugs and Biologics. Guidance for Industry.* Center for Biologics Evaluation and Research (CBER); 2019.

6. U.S. Food and Drug Administration. *Adaptive Designs for Medical Device Clinical Studies Guidance for Industry and Food and Drug Administration Staff.* United States Department of Health and Human Services; 2016.

7. Hummel J, Wang S, Kirkpatrick J. Using simulation to optimize adaptive trial designs: applications in learning and confirmatory phase trials. *Clin Investig.* 2015;**5**(4):401–13.

8. Gaydos B, Anderson KM, Berry D, et al. Good practices for adaptive clinical trials in pharmaceutical product development. *Drug Inf J.* 2009;**43**(5):539–56.

9. Thorlund K, Golchi S, Haggstrom J, Mills E. Highly Efficient Clinical Trials Simulator

(HECT): software application for planning and simulating platform adaptive trials. *Gates Open Res.* 2019;**3**:780.

10. Thorlund K, Haggstrom J, Park JJ, Mills EJ. Key design considerations for adaptive clinical trials: a primer for clinicians. *BMJ.* 2018;**360**:k698.

11. Wason JM, Brocklehurst P, Yap C. When to keep it simple–adaptive designs are not always useful. *BMC Med.* 2019;**17**(1):1–7.

12. Thall P, Fox P, Wathen J. Statistical controversies in clinical research: scientific and ethical problems with adaptive randomization in comparative clinical trials. *Ann Oncol.* 2015;**26**(8):1621–8.

13. Meyer EL, Mesenbrink P, Mielke T, et al. Systematic review of available software for multi-arm multi-stage and platform clinical trial design. *Trials.* 2021;**22**(1):183.

14. Weston SJ, Yee D. Why you should become a useR: a brief introduction to R. *APS Obs.* 2017;**30**(3).

15. Grayling MJ, Wason JM. A web application for the design of multi-arm clinical trials. *BMC Cancer.* 2020;**20**(1):80.

16. Wassmer G, Pahlke F. Rpact: confirmatory adaptive clinical trial design and analysis. R package version; 2021.

17. Kunzmann K, Pilz M, Herrmann C, Rauch G, Kieser M. The adoptr package: adaptive optimal designs for clinical trials in R. *J Stat Softw.* 2021;**98**:1–21.

18. Granholm A, Jensen AKG, Lange T, Kaas-Hansen BS. adaptr: an R package for simulating and comparing adaptive clinical trials. *J Open Source Softw.* 2022;**7**(72):4284.

Characteristics and Principles of Master Protocols

6

Jay J. H. Park, J. Kyle Wathen, and Edward J. Mills

Key Points of This Chapter

In this chapter, we discuss the key concepts, terminologies, and principles of master protocols. The key points of this chapter are:

- The term 'master protocol' is often misunderstood and misused. This term refers to a single overarching protocol document that is developed with the intention of evaluating multiple interventional hypotheses. Master protocol itself does not refer to a specific type of clinical trial.

- There are three types of clinical trials that are conducted using the master protocol framework: platform trials, basket trials, and umbrella trials.

- While master protocols can naturally extend to adaptive trial designs, the use of adaptive trial designs is not a defining feature of master protocols nor of platform, basket, and umbrella trials.

- Master protocols implement common screening, trial systems, and standardised operating procedures across multiple trial institutions under one centralised governance model. In addition to statistical efficiencies, operational efficiencies can be gained by adopting the master protocol framework.

Introduction

The focus of this chapter is the concept and framework of master protocols for clinical trial research. The term 'master protocol' generally refers to a single overarching protocol developed to answer multiple research questions [1–3]. Master protocols aim to improve coordination and harmonisation of clinical trial research by establishing a common trial infrastructure that can answer multiple interventions with shared operational and design features. Conducting two-arm clinical trials is the most common approach to clinical trial research. These trials serve a single purpose of answering whether the single experimental intervention can offer benefit over standard-of-care or placebo [4]. Our discussion up to this point has been on how adaptive trial designs and simulation-guided trial designs can help mitigate areas of inefficiencies in fixed sample size trial designs. Even if the trial is thoughtfully designed and executed, conducting clinical trials with a single purpose can result inefficiencies and duplicated research efforts. As there are usually multiple therapeutic candidates in a given research area, single-purpose clinical trials can result in multiple, independent trials being conducted with redundant trial infrastructure being created for only short-term evaluation. Since these clinical trials are designed by different investigators, they often have inconsistencies in trial and analytical procedures that can create additional challenges when trying to determine what the best intervention option may be for a given disease across multiple trials [5].

The development of master protocols was driven by similar motivation as adaptive enrichment designs and other types of adaptive trial designs that were developed for precision oncology. At inception, the work towards master protocols was motivated and driven to make progress towards the precision medicine movement to identify those therapies that can specifically target cancers based on their genetic make-up [1, 6]. As it is unrealistic to investigate the broad spectrum of multiple genetic sub-populations under the traditional approaches, the master protocol framework has been developed to provide a means to evaluate targeted therapies for precision oncology in a coordinated, efficient, and sustainable manner [6, 7]. There are important key differences between master protocols and adaptive trial designs that are generally misunderstood and misused in the literature [3, 4, 8]. The master protocol framework aims to avoid duplicated efforts and redundancies in clinical trial research overall, whereas adaptive trial designs have initially been developed to improve statistical efficiencies and ethics considerations within each clinical trial.

In this chapter, we discuss the key concepts and terminologies of master protocols including the three types of clinical trials: platform trials, basket trials, and umbrella trials, which are conducted using the master protocol framework. Since first introduced in the form of a peer-reviewed publication in 2015 [6], there have been several inconsistent reporting and usage of the terms 'master protocol', 'platform trial', 'basket trial', and 'umbrella trial' [3]. In this book, we use the definitions used by the U.S. Food and Drug Administration (FDA) given their regulatory oversight and influence of clinical trial research worldwide [1, 9, 10]. We introduce the FDA's definitions and make important distinctions between common terminologies that are used in conjunction with master protocols. We conclude this chapter by discussing the key principles of master protocols that readers should consider in their areas of research.

Important Concepts and Terminologies of Master Protocols

Glossary

- **Basket trial** refers to a clinical trial conducted to test one or more targeted therapies on multiple diseases that share common molecular alternations or other predictive risk factors.
- **Master protocol** (synonym: core protocol, living protocol, or a platform protocol) refers a single overarching protocol developed with the intention of evaluating multiple intervention hypotheses. The term 'master protocol' refers to protocol documents that outline clinical trial procedures and plans for basket, platform, and umbrella trials.
- **Platform trial** refers to a clinical trial that allows addition of new interventions that were not pre-specified in the design stage. Traditionally, clinical trials are limited to one or more interventions that were pre-specified in the design stage.
- **Umbrella trial** refers to a clinical trial that tests two or more targeted therapies for a single disease that is stratified into multiple groups.

Motivation for Master Protocols

With advances in molecular and genomic analyses, there has been increasing calls to use molecular classifications of diseases as a new or complementary disease taxonomy to traditional International Classification of Diseases (ICD) codes that rely on clinical features [11]. Traditional classification of diseases is often based on clinical evaluation and other traditional diagnoses measures, such as histology that involves the examination of cells and tissues using a microscope. Molecular classification of disease, on the other hand, uses genetic and other biomarkers that may reveal information on clinical course and therapeutic responses to potential targeted therapies [12, 13]. Under the molecular classification, multiple diseases under the traditional ICD classifications may be combined into a common molecular disease, or molecular sub-types of traditional disease may be explored for potential targeted therapies.

At inception, the concept of master protocols was largely driven in the United States by the precision oncology movement that relied on molecular classifications of tumours based on their genetic make-up [6, 14–16]. The key stakeholder organisations across the United States included the National Cancer Institute (NCI) of the National Institutes of Health (NIH), FDA, and industry [1, 6, 10, 12]. In May 2018, the NIH launched their 'All of Us' Initiative that aims to gather demographic and biological data from at least 1 million people living in the United States to be used for precision care in oncology and other areas of medicine [17]. In September 2018, the FDA released its draft guidance document on master protocols outlining their recommendations to industry partners for oncology, highlighting their support for a wider dissemination of these master protocols [10]. The FDA has since released its final guidance on master protocols for oncology in 2022 [9], but the release of draft guidance in 2018 should highlight their early role in master protocol methodological development. Between 2009 and 2019, a landscape analysis using a comprehensive literature search has found a rapidly increasing number of the 'master protocol' studies that were largely done by industry [2]. The Clinical Trials Transformation Initiative (CTTI), a public-private partnership co-founded by Duke University and the FDA, has developed resources in 2021 aimed to guide the appropriate use of master protocols, including nomenclature documents, lessons learned, and other useful materials for collaborating on, communicating about, and designing master protocol studies [18].

The motivation for master protocols came from the fact that conducting clinical trials became much more complicated and costly. With increased emphasis on targeted therapies aimed at a sub-type of a disease based on the traditional diagnosis of a disease or a molecular-defined disease population [1, 6, 12], there was a need to coordinate clinical trial research efforts [3]. Recruiting patients with genetic molecular sub-type of one disease, such as cancer patients harbouring a certain mutation of interest, is considerably more difficult than just recruiting all-comers cancer patients [1]. Conducting clinical trials aimed at a molecularly defined disease population requires common trial procedures for biospecimen collection and molecular analysis to confirm eligibility. In addition to complexities associated with molecular screening and recruitment, the calls to improve the efficiency and sustainability of clinical trial research have been motivated the methodological development of master protocols.

Terminologies

The application of innovative trial methods related to master protocols continues to increase, but there has been a lack of standardisation and inconsistency of master protocol

Table 6.1 FDA definitions of master protocol, platform trial, basket trial, and umbrella trial

Term	Definitions
Master protocol	'… [A] protocol designed with multiple substudies, which may have different objectives and [involve] coordinated efforts to evaluate one or more investigational drugs in one or more disease subtypes within the overall trial structure.'
Platform trial	'[A trial designed to] study multiple targeted therapies in the context of a single disease in a perpetual manner, with therapies allowed to enter or leave the platform on the basis of a decision algorithm.'
Basket trial	'A master protocol designed to test a single investigational drug or drug combination in different populations defined by disease stage, histology, number of prior therapies, genetic or other biomarkers, or demographic characteristics.'
Umbrella trial	'A master protocol designed to evaluate multiple investigational drugs administered as single drugs or as drug combinations in a single disease population.'

Note: The definitions presented here were taken from the FDA Draft and Final Guidance on Efficient Clinical Trial Designs and Woodcock et al. 2017 [1, 9, 10].

nomenclatures in the published literature [2, 3, 7]. To facilitate consistent communication, methodological application, and regulatory procedures, it is important to standardise the master protocol nomenclature. While some may disagree, the definitions of master protocols, platform trials, basket trials, and umbrella trials presented by the FDA reflect those that will be used by U.S. and international research industry (Table 6.1). This is reflected by the fact that the 2017 editorial that Woodcock and LaVange, who were directors of the Center for Drug Evaluation and Research (CDER) at the time, published in the *New England Journal of Medicine*, is the most cited paper among the master protocol literature [1].

Platform trials, basket trials, and umbrella trials are three common classifications of clinical trials that are conducted using the master protocol framework [1]. The topic of platform trials is discussed more extensively in Chapter 7, and in Chapter 8 basket and umbrella trials are discussed in more depth. In brief, platform trials refer to clinical trials that allow for new interventions that were not available initially at the design stage to be introduced into the clinical trial [4, 19, 20]. Basket trials refer to clinical trials conducted to test one or more targeted therapies on multiple diseases that share common molecular alternations or other predictive risk factors; umbrella trials refer to clinical trials that test two or more targeted therapies for a single disease that is stratified into multiple groups [2, 3, 8].

In 2019, Siden et al. [3] performed a comprehensive literature search to identify different definitions of master protocols and their sub-types. Considerable variations and inconsistencies in how different clinical trials self-classified themselves as using the master protocol framework. The trials themselves commonly referred to master protocol as being a clinical trial itself. Not surprisingly, the definitions of basket and umbrella trials tended to be more biomarker-focused and oncology-specific. For instance, 77% of the definitions identified in the review for both basket trials ($n = 27/35$) and umbrella trials ($n = 20/26$) used oncology-specific language that limits the scope to one field [3]. In terms of the identified definitions specific to platform trials, while not limited to oncology, some used features of response adaptive randomisation as a defining feature of platform trials [3]. This is even though response adaptive randomisation can be applied to conventional (non-platform) trials that do not allow new interventions to be added.

As we have seen recently with pandemic research related to COVID-19, the master protocol framework can be applied outside of oncology and can bring important efficiency and coordination to answer important interventional related research questions [21, 22]. It is important to use broad definitions that are not restricted to a certain field like oncology to make them widely accessible to a great variety of researchers. Broadening the definitions may also contribute to better adherence and more consistent use of the terminologies. As seen in Table 6.1, the FDA has defined basket trials as having a single intervention, but there are examples of basket trials that allowed for multiple targeted interventions [3]. This issue might be solved by either permitting basket trials to have multiple interventions or by specifying an additional trial type such as a 'multi-basket'. With an understanding that the FDA definitions should continue to be refined, we recommend a cautious adoption of the FDA definitions as standard nomenclatures.

Master Protocols versus Platform, Basket, and Umbrella Trials

In contrast to platform, basket, and umbrella trials, the term 'master protocol' itself does not refer to any specific trial designs [3]. Rather, master protocol refers to a series of protocol documents that is coupled with novel trial designs used in platform, basket, and umbrella trials. A master protocol is used to outline the clinical trial procedures and plans that are updated over time, so others have referred to a master protocol as a 'core protocol', 'living protocol', or a 'platform protocol' [23, 24]. The term has often been misused, and many have used it to describe specific trial designs of platform, basket, and umbrella trials and even adaptive trial designs [3]. However, reader should note that this is a misuse of the term, since a master protocol simply refers to a collection of protocol documents.

Comparison against Adaptive Trial Designs

Clinical trials being conducted using a master protocol framework can be conducted with fixed or adaptive trial designs [9, 10]. It is a misconception that platform, basket, or umbrella trials must be conducted with adaptive trial designs, albeit they are frequently used in these clinical trials [2]. Under the master protocol framework, different sub-studies can be conducted while organised and governed by the established master protocol. Specific adaptive or fixed trial designs with different rules can be implemented to tailor the specific research questions that each sub-study aims to answer. Despite different statistical rules, there will be standardised operating procedures and operational components that will be implemented across different sub-studies. As a general goal, the master protocol framework aims to implement measures to harmonise and standardise key design components and operational aspects to achieve better coordination and sustainability than conducting multiple clinical trials that are designed and conducted independently [1].

Principles of Master Protocols

Common Screening and Trial Systems

Patient recruitment to clinical trials is a well-recognised challenge to any clinical trial research [25]. In biomarker-guided trials, patient recruitment can become difficult, especially when the targeted mechanism of action involves a rare genetic sub-type of a disease [26]. Assessment of eligibility criteria involves collection of a biospecimen from potentially eligible patients and genomic screening (e.g., next-generation DNA sequencing) for target mutation. This can lead to higher rates of screening failure due to only a sub-set of patients harbouring the target mutation. Numbers of genomic test procedures and patients screened will inevitably be greater than number of patients recruited. While the cost of genomic screening has been going down [27], the accumulative total cost of thousands of genomic tests can easily add up to a substantial amount. Having a common screening platform in which multiple biomarker targets can be embedded into a single protocol can result in important screening efficiency and reduction in trial cost, while improving the trial's operational feasibility [1]. A common screening platform can make it easier to provide more visible opportunities to recruit patients into clinical trial research [1, 28, 29]. Harmonisation of trial procedures for genomic screening from sample collection, processing, and analysis can enable high-quality genomic data collection [1, 28, 29]. In addition to common genomic screening and patient recruitment, the use of a central randomisation system and trial database can improve operational efficiency and feasibility. Having centralised systems can shorten start-up times when new interventions or sub-studies are added into the existing trial infrastructure. It can also make the job easier for research coordinators and other site staff performing the day-to-day activities for the trial.

Establishment of Standardised Operating Procedures for Common Trial Infrastructure

In clinical trials, patient screening, recruitment, and other trial procedures often adhere to their own standardised operating procedures (SOPs). SOPs refer to procedural documents with detailed instructions on practices and processes to assure execution of research tasks in accordance with the prepared trial plans. SOPs contain adequate details that act as a guide for research staff through different trial procedures to establish uniformity of day-to-day operational management. Common areas of SOPs include but are not limited to administrative, clinical, data, laboratory, and pharmacy management and procedures in clinical trial research. Different institutions have their own SOPs, and as each institution has different ways of being compliant with regulatory requirements, between clinical trials using different SOPs can have important variations that can potentially hinder data sharing and common analyses from being conducted [30–32].

While the use of SOPs to ensure Good Clinical Practice (GCP) at trial sites is not new, establishment and implementation of common SOPs across multiple sites and multiple interventions is a unique feature of master protocols. Under the master protocol framework, the clinical trials usually establish a large trial network and a common infrastructure established across and through multiple institutions. This is often necessary to ensure that the trial can recruit an adequate number of patients to ensure high statistical power to detect clinically meaningful treatment effects. Across these institutions, implementation of common SOPs can better harmonise clinical trial procedures for screening, recruitment, data collection, patient management, statistical analyses, and more.

By establishing a large trial infrastructure with an increased number of sites and investigators, the master protocol framework aims to create a network effect that can harmonise clinical trial research efforts. This can be exemplified by the role platform trials have had in the therapeutic research for the COVID-19 pandemic. Despite having thousands of clinical trials being registered for COVID-19 research [33, 34], only a handful of platform trials were able to recruit enough patients to produce convincing and actionable clinical trial evidence for patient management [21, 35]. Many of the platform trials conducted for COVID-19 could obtain national-level collaboration and buy-in from major stakeholders. For instance, the UK's four medical officers and the NHS England and NHS Improvement's national medical director publicised a joint letter in May 2020 that encouraged physicians and hospitals to enrol patients into four platform trials (i.e., RECOVERY, ACCORD, PRINCIPLE, and REMAP-CAP) [36]. With such national buy-in and cooperation, the RECOVERY trial was able to rapidly recruit an impressively large number of patients to first generate convincing evidence that supported the use of dexamethasone as a treatment option for hospitalised COVID-19 patients [37].

Centralised Governance and Decision Making

For all clinical trial research, it is generally recommended to adopt a formal governance structure. The composition of different committees involved in trial coordination and conduct should be outlined, with the general membership and their roles and responsibilities clearly identified. Having a formal governance structure helps to ensure that roles and responsibilities of different committees are clearly understood. While such practices are not unique to master protocols, it is important to note that centralised governance for multiple sub-studies that are conducted under the master protocol is an important advantage.

Instead of multiple committees with similar roles and responsibilities being created across multiple independent trials, having common governing committees for all sub-studies can lead to fewer resources. For instance, recruiting statisticians and clinical scientists with experience participating in the Data and Safety Monitoring Board (DSMB) can often be challenging. Having a single DSMB responsible that can monitor the progress of multiple sub-studies and interventions is more efficient than having multiple independent DSMBs, since that will require a larger number of experienced personnel. Similar benefits exist for establishing a common statistical independent analysis centre. Centralised ethics and regulatory review processes are often used for master protocols. This can considerably shorten study start-up time, as adding an intervention into an existing trial can be faster than starting a new trial.

The framework of master protocol can enable multi-stakeholder engagement. It is often recommended to include representations of patient advocates, professional societies, and other consortia who can enable patient-centred decision making and scientific buy-in of the master protocols. In platform and umbrella trials, there are usually multiple industry partners looking to add their experimental therapies for clinical trial evaluation. Centralised decision making on how to prioritise what types of therapies are evaluated in the trial can help ensure that experimental therapies with greater promise and likelihood of patient benefits are prioritised over other therapies.

Use of Adaptive Trial Designs

While the complexities of statistical methods can vary greatly between different types of trials, master protocols are a natural extension of adaptive trial designs. Since these clinical trials often involve evaluation of multiple interventions, adaptive trial designs, particularly sequential designs, can be used to screen out poor performing therapies early. The saved sample size can be diverted to test other experimental therapies instead. Different trials have also used response adaptive randomisation based on ethical reasons [32, 38-43]. However, case-by-case considerations for adaptive trial designs should be made for platform, basket, and umbrella trials.

Secondary Use of Collected Data

Master protocols enable collection of high-quality data, often in large quantity. We can take advantage of coordinated data collection to support other research than just the primary question that the trial is powered to answer. For example, there are examples of trials using master protocols that have aimed to prospectively validate biomarkers for clinical use [41, 44]. As long-term data are often collected from the control group, these trial data can be used to serve the similar purpose as natural history studies to gain a better insight on hallmarks of the disease and how they may progress over time [45]. As secondary analyses, prognostic factors of a given disease and relationships of early surrogate outcomes have been explored [46, 47]. There are many other possibilities for other research questions that are enabled by master protocols.

Conclusion

Early on, the scope of master protocols has largely been limited to oncology. As the principles of master protocols and their sub-types in platform, basket, and umbrella trials can be tailored and adapted for a wide range of health research areas, we are seeing more of these clinical trials being conducted outside of oncology. The advocates of master protocols have included important stakeholders, such as the FDA, that have promoted these clinical trials instead of single-purpose clinical trials. We will likely continue to see increasing numbers of clinical trials being conducted using the master protocol framework. While planning and execution of master protocols can be complicated, such framework can be an effective way to improve the quality and standardisation of trial research while establishing long-term trial infrastructure. Now that we have finished discussing the concept of master protocols in this chapter, we will discuss their sub-types in platform trials in Chapter 7 and basket and umbrella trials in Chapter 8.

References

1. Woodcock J, LaVange LM. Master protocols to study multiple therapies, multiple diseases, or both. *N Eng J Med*. 2017;**377**(1):62–70.

2. Park JJH, Siden E, Zoratti MJ, et al. Systematic review of basket trials, umbrella trials, and platform trials: a landscape analysis of master protocols. *Trials*. 2019;**20**(1):572.

3. Siden EG, Park JJ, Zoratti MJ, et al. Reporting of master protocols towards a standardized approach: a systematic review. *Contemp Clin Trials Commun*. 2019;**15**:100406.

4. Park JJH, Harari O, Dron L, et al. An overview of platform trials with a checklist for clinical readers. *J Clin Epidemiol*. 2020;**125**:1–8.

5. Mills EJ, Thorlund K, Ioannidis JP. Demystifying trial networks and network meta-analysis. *BMJ*. 2013;**346**:f2914.

6. Redman MW, Allegra CJ. The master protocol concept. *Semin Oncol*. 2015;**42**(5):724–30.

7. Hirakawa A, Asano J, Sato H, Teramukai S. Master protocol trials in oncology: review and new trial designs. *Contemp Clin Trials Commun*. 2018;**12**:1–8.

8. Park JJH, Hsu G, Siden EG, Thorlund K, Mills EJ. An overview of precision oncology basket and umbrella trials for clinicians. *CA Cancer J Clin*. 2020;**70**(2):125–37.

9. United States Department of Health and Human Services, Food and Drug Administration. *Master Protocols: Efficient Clinical Trial Design Strategies to Expedite Development of Oncology Drugs and Biologics Guidance for Industry*. United States Department of Health and Human Services; 2022. www.fda.gov/media/120721/download.

10. United States Department of Health and Human Services, Food and Drug Administration. *Master Protocols: Efficient Clinical Trial Design Strategies to Expedite Development of Oncology Drugs and Biologics Guidance for Industry (Draft Guidance)*. United States Department of Health and Human Services; 2018. www.fda.gov/downloads/Drugs/Guidance ComplianceRegulatoryInformation/Guidances/UCM621817.pdf.

11. Zhou X, Lei L, Liu J, et al. A systems approach to refine disease taxonomy by integrating phenotypic and molecular networks. *EBioMedicine*. 2018;**31**:79–91.

12. Mullauer L. Milestones in pathology-from histology to molecular biology. *Memo*. 2017;**10**(1):42–5.

13. Zhang H, Zeng Z, Mukherjee A, Shen B. Molecular diagnosis and classification of inflammatory bowel disease. *Expert Rev Mol Diagn*. 2018;**18**(10):867–86.

14. Abrams J, Conley B, Mooney M, et al. National Cancer Institute's Precision Medicine Initiatives for the new National Clinical Trials Network. *Am Soc Clin Oncol Educ Book*. 2014:71–6.

15. Heckman-Stoddard BM, Smith JJ. Precision medicine clinical trials: defining new treatment strategies. *Semin Oncol Nurs*. 2014;**30**(2):109–16.

16. Kumar-Sinha C, Chinnaiyan AM. Precision oncology in the age of integrative genomics. *Nat Biotechnol*. 2018;**36**(1):46–60.

17. National Institutes of Health All of US Research Program. About the All of Us Research Program. Cited 2019. https://allofus.nih.gov/about/about-all-us-research-program

18. Clinical Trials Transformation Initiative. Master Protocol Studies; 2021 https://ctti-clinicaltrials.org/our-work/novel-clinical-trial-designs/master-protocol-studies/

19. Berry SM, Connor JT, Lewis RJ. The platform trial: an efficient strategy for evaluating multiple treatments. *JAMA*. 2015;**313**(16):1619–20.

20. Adaptive Platform Trials C. Adaptive platform trials: definition, design, conduct and reporting considerations. *Nat Rev Drug Discov*. 2019;**18**(10):797–807.

21. Park JJH, Dron L, Mills EJ. Moving forward in clinical research with master protocols. *Contemp Clin Trials*. 2021;**106**:106438.

22. Vanderbeek AM, Bliss JM, Yin Z, Yap C. Implementation of platform trials in the COVID-19 pandemic: a rapid review. *Contemp Clin Trials*. 2022;**112**:106625.

23. Dean NE, Gsell PS, Brookmeyer R, et al. Creating a framework for conducting randomized clinical trials during disease outbreaks. *N Engl J Med*. 2020;**382**(14):1366–9.

24. Schiavone F, Bathia R, Letchemanan K, et al. This is a platform alteration: a trial management perspective on the operational aspects of adaptive and platform and umbrella protocols. *Trials*. 2019;**20**(1):264.

25. Fogel DB. Factors associated with clinical trials that fail and opportunities for improving the likelihood of success: a review. *Contemp Clin Trials Commun*. 2018;**11**:156–64.

26. Antoniou M, Kolamunnage-Dona R, Wason J, et al. Biomarker-guided trials: challenges in practice. *Contemp Clin Trials Commun*. 2019;**16**:100493.

27. Preston J, VanZeeland A, Peiffer D. Innovation at Illumina: the road to the $600 human genome. *Nature (Illumia)*. 2021.

28. Lam VK, Papadimitrakopoulou V. Master protocols in lung cancer: experience from Lung Master Protocol. *Curr Opin Oncol*. 2018;**30**(2):92–7.

29. Ferrarotto R, Redman MW, Gandara DR, Herbst RS, Papadimitrakopoulou VA.

Lung-MAP – framework, overview, and design principles. *Chin Clin Oncol.* 2015;**4**(3):36.

30. Houston L, Yu P, Martin A, Probst Y. Heterogeneity in clinical research data quality monitoring: a national survey. *J Biomed Inform.* 2020;**108**:103491.

31. Kuchinke W, Ohmann C, Yang Q, et al. Heterogeneity prevails: the state of clinical trial data management in Europe – results of a survey of ECRIN centres. *Trials.* 2010;**11**:79.

32. Remap-Cap Investigators, ACTIV-4a Investigators, Attacc Investigators, Goligher EC, Bradbury CA, McVerry BJ, et al. Therapeutic anticoagulation with heparin in critically ill patients with Covid-19. *N Engl J Med.* 2021;**385** (9):777–89.

33. Thorlund K, Dron L, Park J, et al. A real-time dashboard of clinical trials for COVID-19. *Lancet Digit Health.* 2020;**2**(6): e286–e7.

34. Dillman A, Park JJH, Zoratti MJ, et al. Reporting and design of randomized controlled trials for COVID-19: a systematic review. *Contemp Clin Trials.* 2021;**101**:106239.

35. Park JJ, Mogg R, Smith GE, et al. How COVID-19 has fundamentally changed clinical research in global health. *Lancet Glob Health.* 2021;**9**(5):e711–e20.

36. NIHR. Recruiting patients for clinical trials for COVID-19 therapeutics. 2020. www .nihr.ac.uk/news/uks-chief-medical-officers-urge-hospitals-to-recruit-60-of-eligible-covid-19-patients-into-recovery-trial/25515

37. Recovery Collaborative Group, Horby P, Lim WS, Emberson JR, et al. Dexamethasone in hospitalized patients with Covid-19. *N Engl J Med.* 2021;**384** (8):693–704.

38. Berry DA, Graves T, Connor J, et al. Adaptively randomized seamless-phase multiarm platform trial: Glioblastoma Multiforme Adaptive Global Innovative Learning Environment (GBM AGILE). *Cancer Research.* 2017;**77**(13 Supplement 1).

39. Rugo HS, Olopade OI, DeMichele A, et al. Adaptive randomization of veliparib-carboplatin treatment in breast cancer. *N Eng J Med.* 2016;**375**(1):23–34.

40. Barker AD, Sigman CC, Kelloff GJ, et al. I-SPY 2: an adaptive breast cancer trial design in the setting of neoadjuvant chemotherapy. *Clin Pharmacol Ther.* 2009;**86**(1):97–100.

41. Papadimitrakopoulou V, Lee JJ, Wistuba, II, et al. The BATTLE-2 study: a biomarker-integrated targeted therapy study in previously treated patients with advanced non-small-cell lung cancer. *J Clin Oncol.* 2016;**34**(30):3638–47.

42. Tam AL, Kim ES, Lee JJ, et al. Feasibility of image-guided transthoracic core-needle biopsy in the BATTLE lung trial. *J Thorac Oncol.* 2013;**8**(4):436–42.

43. Kim ES, Herbst RS, Wistuba, II, et al. The BATTLE trial: personalizing therapy for lung cancer. *Cancer Discov.* 2011;**1** (1):44–53.

44. Wang H, Yee D. I-SPY 2: a neoadjuvant adaptive clinical trial designed to improve outcomes in high-risk breast cancer. *Curr Breast Cancer Rep.* 2019;**11**(4):303–10.

45. Bogin V. Master protocols: new directions in drug discovery. *Contemp Clin Trials Commun.* 2020;**18**:100568.

46. Ali A, Hoyle A, Haran AM, et al. Association of bone metastatic burden with survival benefit from prostate radiotherapy in patients with newly diagnosed metastatic prostate cancer: a secondary analysis of a randomized clinical trial. *JAMA Oncol.* 2021;**7**(4):555–63.

47. Cortazar P, Geyer CE. Pathological complete response in neoadjuvant treatment of breast cancer. *Ann Surg Oncol.* 2015;**22**(5):1441–6.

Platform Trials

Jay J. H. Park, J. Kyle Wathen, and Edward J. Mills

Key Points of This Chapter

In this chapter, we discuss the terminology of platform trials and their key design considerations. The key points of this chapter are:

- Platform trials refer to clinical trials that allow new interventions to be added to the platform over time even if they are not pre-specified in the design stage. Platform trials can be applied to all phases of clinical trial research. While they are most often conducted as randomised clinical trials with adaptive trial designs (adaptive platform randomised trials), they can be conducted with non-randomised or fixed sample trial designs as well.

- As a general goal, platform trials aim to establish a shared trial infrastructure in which multiple interventions can be evaluated. Conducting a single platform trial can help avoid independent clinical trial evaluations being conducted by multiple separate teams with shorter term infrastructure and trials that would otherwise compete against each other.

- Platform trials represent an exciting turning point for clinical research. The key design considerations of platform trials are outlined in this chapter.

Introduction to Platform Trials

There has been increasing interest in platform trials that has led to important methodological advancements towards platform trial designs in a considerably short amount of time [1]. While most platform trials have taken place for oncology prior to the COVID-19 pandemic [2], they have become much more popular and common during the pandemic because platform trials have played important roles in therapeutics for COVID-19 [3, 4]. We expect the use of platform trials will continue to increase, so it is important that we discuss key characteristics of platform trials and their key design considerations in this chapter.

Platform trials refer to a type of clinical trial in which new interventions that were not pre-specified in the initial design stage are to be added into the ongoing trial [5–7]. They are designed to permit evaluation of multiple interventions in a perpetual manner using a single master protocol that establishes a common trial infrastructure with standardised operating procedures and often with the same statistical analysis plan. The established platform acts as a single, common infrastructure wherein interventions can be added and discontinued at different times as their clinical questions are answered over time [5–7]. Often, they are conducted as randomised clinical trials with adaptive trial designs, but they can be conducted as non-randomised, fixed sample trial designs [2]. The randomised platform trials

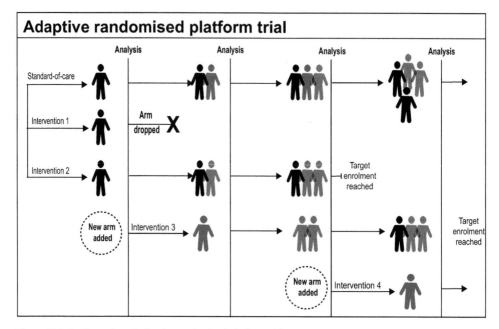

Figure 7.1 An illustration of adaptive randomised platform trial.

This is an illustrative example of a platform trial that starts with three study arms including a common control arm that consists of standard-of-care. For each study arm, the platform trial is planned for three statistical analyses. At the first analysis, Intervention 1 is dropped while a new arm (Intervention 3) is introduced into the platform. At the third analysis, enrolment to Intervention 2 is stopped after meeting its enrolment target, and another intervention (Intervention 4) is added. At the fourth analysis, enrolment to Intervention 3 is stopped again due to meeting its enrolment target. This hypothetical trial perpetually continues with the control arm and Intervention 4.

allow for multiple interventions to be simultaneously evaluated against a common control group [5–7]. In addition to being designed with the flexibility of allowing new interventions to be added over time, the control group and the standard-of-care provided can be updated during the trial, as interventions are shown to be effective or ineffective over time [7]. Platform trials with adaptive trial designs (adaptive platform trials) also include pre-specified plans that allow the trial to respond to accumulating trial data, with sequential designs being commonly used to allow an intervention to stop early based on futility or success [7, 8] (Figure 7.1).

Motivation for Platform Trials

Most clinical trials are conducted as two-arm trials [9]. Two-arm trials serve a single purpose of answering whether the experimental intervention being studied can offer benefit over the standard-of-care or placebo that is included as the competing control arm. Conducting two-arm trials can be inefficient, since this can result in multiple independent trials requiring competing infrastructure for each short-term evaluation and more patients being random-ised to placebo or standard-of-care compared to having a single platform trial [10]. There are, of course, multi-arm trials with a wider scope, but they still lack the flexibility to fully overcome the limitations of two-arm trials, particularly in research areas where frequent therapeutic discoveries are made [11, 12]. Conventionally, these trials have a defined end and only compare pre-specified intervention(s). If a therapeutic discovery is made after a clinical trial begins, regardless of whether they are two-arm or multi-arm trials, a new trial may be needed to determine its efficacy [12]. Even with multi-arm studies, the scope of their clinical evaluation can largely remain focused on a few interventions ('intervention-focused designs').

Intervention-focused approaches can result in multiple, independent trials being conducted with redundant infrastructures being created for shorter-term evaluation and a larger number of patients being randomised to standard-of-care or placebo [13-15]. These trials often have different, non-standardised trial data collection and analysis procedures, so there are additional challenges when trying to determine what may be the best intervention option for a given condition across multiple trials [16]. Instead of these clinical trials being conducted with 'intervention-focused' designs, platform trials can be much more 'disease-focused' [17]. They allow for evaluation of multiple interventions, even those that were not available at the start of the trial, in a perpetual manner while being adaptable for both internal and external scientific discoveries. If the internal trial data show that one of the interventions being studied is superior to the control, that intervention can become a new control. The platform trial can also adapt when an external trial demonstrates that one of the interventions being evaluated in the platform is beneficial [18, 19]. The nature of platform trials can thus be described as disease-focused trials that can ultimately answer the question, 'What is the best intervention option for a given disease?' [17]. Platform trials can thus have important advantages over intervention-focused designs (e.g., two-arm trials), especially in settings where multiple competing but unestablished treatments with new treatments on the horizon.

Response to COVID-19

In response to novel coronavirus disease 2019 (COVID-19), billions of dollars in research and development (R&D) funding have been invested to rapidly discover treatment and preventive measures against the disease. When COVID-19 has become a singular focus for the scientific community during the pandemic, we have observed inefficiencies of the clinical trial enterprise [20, 21]. There have been thousands of clinical trials with predominantly two-arm trial designs that had been registered for COVID-19. Yet, there have been arguably only a handful of clinical trials (e.g., Randomised Evaluation of COVID-19 Therapy [RECOVERY], SOLIDARITY, Randomized, Embedded, Multifactorial Adaptive Platform Trial for Community-Acquired Pneumonia [REMAP-CAP], TOGETHER, Accelerating COVID-19 Therapeutic Interventions and Vaccines [ACTIV], and Platform Randomised Trial of Treatments in the Community for Epidemic and Pandemic illnesses [PRINCIPLE]) that generated actional evidence for COVID-19 [22-27]. These trials share a common characteristic of being a platform randomised trial governed by a master protocol that allowed for evaluation of multiple interventions including many that were not pre-specified in the beginning. Platform trials have demonstrated important advantages compared to traditional intervention-focused designs for COVID-19, a setting outside oncology during the COVID-19 pandemic [4, 8, 28].

Characteristics of Platform Trials

Shared Infrastructure and Evaluation of Multiple Interventions

Different platform trials will vary in design and objectives, but there are important shared characteristics. They all try to reduce redundancy in trial efforts and resources by establishing a shared infrastructure in which multiple interventions can be evaluated. Platform trials permit evaluation of multiple different interventions in a shared trial infrastructure with common design elements and standardised operating procedures. In many platform trials, a large trial network can be established across multiple trial centres using standardised operating procedures outlined in the master protocol [1, 5]. Coordinated screening mechanisms with centralised trial systems are implemented to streamline and improve the quality of many trial processes and logistics [5]. The common database(s) and randomisation system across the shared infrastructure may allow for more seamless integration of the new interventions being added into the trial. These features combined with centralised analytics may improve standardisation of clinical evaluation and reporting of different interventions being evaluated in the platform over time. Otherwise, independent evaluation of interventions would require multiple separate teams creating separate protocols, recruiting participating centres, establishing a methods centre, obtaining ethics approval, and addressing all the challenges that arise as the trial proceeds. Conducting multiple trials independently could result in inefficiencies. Within a platform trial, these efforts are mostly done once and harmonised to reduce redundancy in efforts [1, 5].

Platform randomised trials can improve efficiency by reducing the number of patients needed in the control group compared with the numbers of participants that would be needed in multiple independent randomised clinical trials [6, 29]. Such sample size savings represent an efficiency that could allow testing of more interventions than in multiple, separate intervention trials. The efficiencies could result in lower costs relative to multiple individual trials that address the same questions, addressing more interventions with the same cost, or some combination [11]. When effective interventions are identified in a platform trial, the control and standard-of-care can be updated in the platform, allowing research to continue towards investigating additional improvement in the new standard-of-care.

Adaptive Trial Designs of Platform Trials

Adaptive platform randomised trials are the most common type of platform trials [2]. As a result, they have been referred to as an extension of adaptive trial designs, called multi-arm, multi-stage (MAMS) designs, since multiple interventions (multi-arm) undergoing multiple interim analyses (multi-stage) are often part of their design features. In contrast to MAMS design, it is important to note that platform trials have the additional flexibilities of allowing new experimental arms to be added and the control arm to be updated during the trial [1, 2, 5, 6, 30]. They allow for multiple interventions to be evaluated in a perpetual manner under a single protocol that establishes common design elements [1, 2, 5, 6, 30].

Well-planned adaptive platform trials will use statistical analyses with pre-specified adaptations and decision rules. Adaptive platform trials most commonly use sequential designs that will allow for early stopping for futility and/or efficacy [1, 2]. Similar to other clinical trials that allow early stopping at a pre-specified interim analysis, efficacy and statistical superiority thresholds for early stopping are generally chosen to be more conservative for interim analyses than the final analysis of trials that continue to completion, as the accuracy of treatment effect estimates in trials that are stopped early for efficacy can be a concern when the sample size is small [31, 32]. Response adaptive randomisation is a potential design feature in multi-intervention platform trials in which allocation ratios can be adapted, based on pre-specified rules, at each interim analysis over the course of the trial [33, 34]. The allocation ratio among the intervention groups is adapted to favour the interventions with more favourable interim results, while keeping the allocation ratio to the control group fixed [33, 34].

As each platform trial will have different goals and therefore design features, there are no default interim analyses plans that are best for all platform trials, and the simulations should be conducted before starting the trial to determine the best design for each platform trial [35]. The process of simulating virtual patients in virtual trial designs is used to inform, revise, and determine the final statistical design including the interim analyses plans and decision rules. Many of the adaptive design features can affect the performance characteristics of a given platform trial. Therefore, it is important to evaluate different design features during the planning stage [31, 36].

Comparison versus Basket and Umbrella Trials

Platform trials, basket trials, and umbrella trials are three types of clinical trials that can be conducted under the master protocol framework [2, 5, 37]. In basket trials, a targeted therapy is evaluated for multiple diseases with a common risk factor, such as a molecular alteration, or risk factors that that may help predict whether patients will respond to the given therapy. Umbrella trials evaluate multiple targeted therapies in a single disease that is stratified into multiple sub-studies based on different molecular or other predictive risk factors [1, 5, 37]. Basket and umbrella trials refer to specific types of clinical trials conducted to evaluate targeted therapies. Both basket and umbrella trials can be platform trials in nature if they are designed to allow for the addition of new interventions during the trial [7].

Key Design Considerations of Platform Trials

Estimands

In Chapter 1, we discussed the framework of estimands. Most clinical trials aim to draw a conclusion about the treatment effect in a specific population as a primary goal. An estimand refers to such target quantity of treatment that the trial aims to measure and estimate from the data collected in the trial [38]. Implementation of the estimand framework is critical for trial planning. This has been discussed extensively for conventional (non-platform) trials, but it is not as clear for platform trials where multiple interventions will be evaluated [39]. In most clinical trials, we usually establish a single primary estimand for a single treatment, but this may not be desirable for platform trials, where multiple interventions will be evaluated. This is not to say platform trials and other complex trials are an exception of setting clear trial objectives and estimands at the design stage [39]. For multiple interventions, including those that cannot be anticipated for in the design stage, it might be desirable to set different estimands for different therapies [39].

In most platform trials that have been conducted thus far, it has been a common practice to use a single primary estimand for different interventions [2]. In other words, interventions, regardless of when they are added to the platform, would be evaluated using a pre-specified analysis plan with the same primary endpoint and strategy for intercurrent events, as outlined in the protocol documents [2]. Once the master protocol is finalised, new interventions would follow the pre-specified plans for statistical analyses including the same interim analyses and decision rules. This is done so that there are few deviations from the master protocols, even in an evolving clinical field during an ongoing platform trial.

It is possible for platform trials to have multiple objectives and therefore multiple primary estimands between different interventions. This will require some careful considerations. Not all estimands can easily be defined at the start of the trial, but the primary estimand should be defined when a new intervention is added. The decision on the choice of the primary estimand should be based on scientific merits and not based on knowledge of unblinded trial data. There should be a centralised governance and process in place to determine which drug should be considered in the platform and how the drug should be evaluated. The practice of choosing the estimand based on knowledge of the unblinded trial data should be prevented. In platform trials, it is common for data to be shared across different statistical comparisons, such as having a shared control arm that multiple interventions will be evaluated against. This will require a pre-defined core set of outcomes and other data variables (e.g., covariates to be used in the analyses) in the protocol and the case report forms (CRFs). As new interventions are added to the platform, new changes from the master protocol can be pre-specified in their intervention-specific appendix or sub-protocol. However, the goal should be to have as few deviations from the master protocol as possible.

Estimators

Platform trials are designed to evaluate multiple interventions in a single trial, so there are multiple hypotheses that will be tested. As in the case of pre-specifying the estimand, it is important to pre-specify how each estimand will be estimated. Statistical analysis plan should be clearly identified including the detailed plans for the primary analysis and interim analysis plan if adaptive trial designs will be used. Such details are usually presented in the main statistical analysis plan with an adaptive trial design report outlining the simulation approach and results. In platform trials, pairwise comparisons between each of the intervention arms versus the control arm are often used as the primary analysis. When the primary comparisons are versus the control, sample size calculations are performed accordingly, where the desired statistical properties for detecting an effect (e.g., 80% power and 5% type I error rate) apply to each analysis. In such case, each intervention arm will have the same recruitment target when the trial is initiated and when a new intervention arm is introduced because the desired treatment effect is the same for all control comparisons.

Interim Analysis Plans

Careful consideration of interim analysis plans for adaptive platform trials is needed. This is similar to conventional (non-platform) trials using adaptive trial designs. It is important to consider the frequency and timing of interim analyses, as well as outcomes and decision rules that will be used to make the pre-specified adaptations. The frequency of interim evaluations is an important consideration because the risk of false findings can increase along with the number of analyses, especially without adequate statistical adjustments. In adaptive platform trials that allow for the dropping of intervention arms early, conducting interim analyses without adjustments can increase the risk of dropping effective arms and inflating the risk for false negative findings [33, 36]. In other platform trials that allow for early stopping for superiority, it is important to control for potential inflation in false positive rates [33, 36]. In terms of timing of an interim analysis, it is particularly important to consider when the first interim analysis will be conducted. Making an interim evaluation too early can be problematic, as small datasets are more prone to random error [33, 36]. As with all trials that employ interim evaluations, platform trials need an appropriately sized 'burn-in period', where enough data can be collected to allow for reasonable precision such that erroneous decisions to drop an intervention arm can be avoided [33, 36]. The details of the interim analyses, including the frequency, timing, and burn-in period, are often determined using trial simulations. As discussed in Chapter 5, simulations should be done on a variety of factors, such as the duration of interventions and follow-up, the recruitment target and rate, and expected treatment effects [36].

As in all adaptive clinical trials, the choice of outcomes for interim analyses is critical for platform trials. In a given trial, the outcome used for the final analysis is the primary question of interest (primary outcome). If the primary outcome is quick to observe and/or is simple to measure, platform trials likely will not use two separate outcomes for the interim analyses and the final analysis. In instances in which the primary outcome is slow to observe and/or invasive, a surrogate outcome that is quicker or simpler to measure may be used for interim evaluations (intermediate outcome) [40]. Between the primary and intermediate outcomes, there should be a strong clinical justification that an improvement in the intermediate outcome should lead to an improvement in the primary outcome, and vice versa [14, 40].

The use of an intermediate outcome can potentially provide an efficient way to screen interventions, but this is dependent on the choice of intermediate outcome [41, 42]. The choice in the intermediate outcome is appropriate if it has a strong association with the primary outcome [41, 42]. For example, research suggests that progression-free survival is highly correlated with overall survival for patients with previously treated chronic lympho-cytic leukaemia [43]. In contrast, the same relationship between these outcomes is not always observed in other tumour types (e.g., metastatic breast cancer) [44] or for specific treatment classes [45]. Careful consideration is warranted on a case-by-case basis for the relationship between such outcomes. If the improvements in the intermediate outcome do not translate to improved primary outcome, the choice in the intermediate outcome will be erroneous. An erroneous choice in the intermediate outcome may lead to erroneous findings that may result in 'effective' interventions not being selected for the final evalu-ation, or 'ineffective' interventions being selected.

Statistical criteria used to drop or graduate intervention arms onto the next stage are referred to as decision rules [33, 36]. The choice of decision rules is important for platform trials to minimise the risk of biased and even inefficient decision making regarding the interim evaluations. Decision rules can be based on both frequentist and Bayesian statistical metrics [31, 33, 46-48]. Platform trials are neither strictly Bayesian nor frequentist. They can be conducted using both statistical frameworks. There are no default decision rules for platform trials, as each trial may have different design features and goals for clinical evaluation. In the planning stage, extensive simulations are usually conducted in order to establish decision rules that minimise statistical error rates and optimise trial efficiency (e.g., time, sample size, and patient exposure to inferior arms) [31, 49, 50]. These decision rules are pre-specified before the first patient is enrolled into the trial and before a new sub-study becomes active in an ongoing platform [29, 31, 49].

Active Number of Interventions

It is often a good idea to pre-specify a maximum number of arms that can be active at a given time simultaneously for operational and feasibility reasons. The number of active arms allowed should be determined with the operational team [51, 52]. As the number of active arms increases, the trial management will become much more difficult. Recruitment challenges such as difficulty in providing patients sufficient information without information overload can be magnified as well [14]. At a given recruitment rate, increasing the number of active arms may lengthen the time required for recruitment targets to be met. For instance, if 50 patients per month can feasibly be recruited and a sample size of 200 patients per arm is required, increasing the number of arms from 4 to 8 will result in an increase in recruitment duration from 16 to 32 months. As larger numbers of active arms are allowed for platform trials, challenges associated with data management and maintenance of intervention supplies can be amplified [51, 52].

In platform trials, the number of arms active for recruitment can vary over time. Contrasted to conventional trials, especially with fixed-sample designs, clinical evaluations of interventions can finish at different times since an intervention may be dropped (i.e., no more participants are randomised to the arm) after an interim evaluation. New intervention arms will finish their trial evaluation later since they are added later. For each arm, it is important to consider the time period that it was active for recruitment and the potential temporal variability. When control arm data are outside of this period, it is important to consider the validity of including these data in the analysis.

Allocation

It is important to consider the allocation ratios between the intervention and control groups. When the control comparisons are the primary focus, statistical power can benefit from allocating more participants to the control. For example, the average confidence interval length is minimised by allocating $n\sqrt{t}$ patients to the control arm, where n is the sample size for each of the arms and t is the number of active arms (Dunnett test) [53]. To maximise power in a platform trial with four experimental arms, the allocation ratio of 2:1:1:1:1 may be ideal with the allocation to the control group being $\sqrt{4} = 2$ times higher than the experimental arms.

While allocating too few participants to the control group may result in reduced power, this can be a worthwhile trade-off between power and precision and improved ethics by allocating more participants to promising experimental interventions. There can be ethical advantages with using adaptive trial design features, such as response adaptive randomisation [36, 54]. However, when the primary analysis involves comparison against the control arm, it is important to maintain adequate allocation to the control. By having multiple interventions, the overall allocation to the control arm can be minimised even without response adaptive randomisation. For the right clinical questions, response adaptive randomisation can have important merits, especially in the setting of a platform trial where multiple interventions will be evaluated. Response adaptive randomisation raises both statistical and operational complexities. It is important to note that response adaptive randomisation is not a defining feature for platform trials.

Introduction of New Interventions

In addition to statistical considerations, there are important non-statistical considerations that need to be made when introducing new interventions into platform trials. These include considerations of scientific merits and mechanisms in which new interventions are to be added into an ongoing platform. When a new intervention is available, several scientific and practical considerations may guide the decisions regarding its inclusion in the trial, including a sound rationale, support by a robust biological hypothesis, positive evidence of potential efficacy, adequate safety profile, ease of administration, and low cost [55, 56]. These scientific merits may be reviewed by an independent working group that consists of members from industry, academia, patient advocacy groups, and others with technical expertise, clinical expertise, or both and who are not directly involved in the platform trial. An independent working group can screen and prioritise candidate interventions to be added to the platform trial in instances for which many interventions could be simultaneously evaluated. Platform trials have adopted using pre-specified scientific criteria that can guide what types of interventions are added [55, 56]. Additionally, platform trials require industry partners that are willing to contribute the pharmaceutical agent, as having sufficient availability of the drug is required for trial evaluation [55, 56].

Having a proper mechanism in place for adding new intervention(s) in platform trials is critical to ensure that data collection and other trial operations are not affected [51, 52]. Amendments to the main master protocol, including updates to CRFs and the trial database used to collect and store the trial data, will be needed [52]. Generic CRFs may be used for the baseline and outcome assessments in all participants with intervention-specific CRFs for treatment and toxicity assessments that are relevant for a given intervention. The structure of the trial database should also be designed with flexibility and scalability from the start. Other important considerations will include mechanisms for peer review of new candidate interventions for their scientific merits and review process by the trial's Institutional Review Board (IRB). Independent evaluation of scientific merits may be done by external reviewers, but consideration of investigator enthusiasm for the new intervention arm will also be considered along with dialogue with the funders to financially support the new comparison [51].

Use of Non-concurrent Control Data

In conventional (non-platform) trials, enrolment for all groups included will start at the same time, with statistical comparisons being made with data from the concurrent groups [57]. A concurrent group refers to participants who were enrolled during the same time period as the participants in other study groups. In platform trials, investigational groups enter and finish the trial at different times. For new interventions that are added into the platform later, there will be a set of previously enrolled participants (non-concurrent data). As diseases may change over time and patient populations may drift, it is not possible to be as confident of prognostic balance – the goal of randomisation – as when patients are randomised concurrently to intervention and control. However, they would be enrolled under the same inclusion and exclusion criteria and had endpoint information collected in a consistent manner, even if the control group participants have not been randomised at the same time as each intervention group participant in the platform trial.

It is possible to incorporate all trial data into a single analysis, regardless of whether they were concurrently or non-concurrently enrolled [7]. For instance, it is possible to incorporate non-concurrent control data for the primary analysis. Sharing control information and using the non-concurrent control group data are qualitatively different from supplementing a trial with historical or observational control group data or external clinical trial data, because the participants met the same trial enrolment criteria and data were measured and collected in a consistent environment [58]. While temporal variability may exist in platform trials, because patients are randomised and followed up with the same standardised operating procedures outlined in the master protocol, non-concurrent control group data collected earlier in the platform trial may have minimal temporal variability compared with concurrent control group data. Using the non-concurrent control group data can increase statistical power, and statistical adjustments for temporal variability and other confounders can minimise the effect of prognostic imbalance. However, incorporating the non-concurrent control group data may not ensure prognostic balance in the same way that randomisation does [59].

When designing a platform trial, using non-concurrent data can be advantageous. If this is done, it is important to conduct sensitivity analyses where the data analysis is limited to concurrent data only. Reporting of both types of analyses and for any inconsistency is critical for transparency of the estimator using non-concurrent control. The statistical methods that were applied to incorporate non-concurrent and concurrent control group data. Non-concurrent control group data may be accounted for by model-ling possible temporal variations in the control population [7, 60]. Statistical methods, such as dynamic borrowing methods, use data-driven approaches to determine the amount of information borrowing based on degree of consistency between the non-concurrent and concurrent data [58, 61–63]. These methods borrow the non-concurrent data the most when they are consistent with the concurrent data and borrow less when the data are inconsistent [61]. These statistical methods are beyond the scope of this book, but the readers can refer to the 2014 article by Viele et al. [61] for further discussion on different borrowing techniques.

Communication and Unanticipated Changes

We believe it is a good practice for the protocol to pre-specify the communication plans for the dissemination of trial results after an intervention in the trial is completed and the responsibilities of a committee (e.g., trial steering committee) that may hold the ultimate decision for approving the reporting of results are completed. It is important to recognise that it is natural for scientific questions being asked in the trial to evolve over time given that platform trials generally are planned for the long term. Over time, it is possible for the control and standard-of-care to be updated if there are internal and/or external scientific discoveries. Since platform trials are generally conducted over a long duration, it would be unethical not to update the control arm, even if this cannot be easily planned ahead of time. New unanticipated scientific questions can naturally arise over time with both new internal and even external scientific discoveries. Since a large amount of high-quality data is collected in a standardised manner, platform trials can allow for different types of secondary analyses including those that are unplanned. Given the long-term or ongoing nature of platform trials, it may also be beneficial to conduct additional simulations when more data become available that may either validate or contradict the assumptions that were made during the planning stage [7].

Conclusion

Methodological advancements in platform trials represent a new and exciting turning point for clinical trial research. In this chapter, we have described the key characteristics of platform trials and reviewed key design considerations that can be used to help interpret the reported results from platform trials. It is likely (or at least we hope) that more scientific investigators will conduct platform trials. Therefore, doing so will be important to the scientific literature of platform trials and key design considerations that have been discussed in this chapter.

Platform trials are often conducted with randomised clinical trials with adaptive trial designs. In this context, adaptive platform trials allow simultaneous comparison of multiple intervention groups against a single control group that serves as a common control based on a pre-specified interim analysis plan. The platform trial design enables introduction of new interventions after the trial is initiated to evaluate multiple interventions in an ongoing manner using a single overarching protocol called a master (or core) protocol. When multiple treatment candidates are available, rapid scientific therapeutic discoveries may be made. Platform trials have important potential advantages in creating an efficient trial infrastructure that can help address critical clinical questions as the evidence evolves.

References

1. Siden EG, Park JJ, Zoratti MJ, et al. Reporting of master protocols towards a standardized approach: a systematic review. *Contemp Clin Trials Commun.* 2019;15:100406.

2. Park JJH, Siden E, Zoratti MJ, et al. Systematic review of basket trials, umbrella trials, and platform trials: a landscape analysis of master protocols. *Trials.* 2019;20 (1):572.

3. Vanderbeek AM, Bliss JM, Yin Z, Yap C. Implementation of platform trials in the COVID-19 pandemic: a rapid review. *Contemp Clin Trials.* 2022;112:106625.

4. Park JJ, Mogg R, Smith GE, et al. How COVID-19 has fundamentally changed clinical research in global health. *Lancet Glob Health.* 2021;9(5):e711–e20.

5. Woodcock J, LaVange LM. Master protocols to study multiple therapies, multiple diseases, or both. *N Eng J Medi.* 2017;377(1):62–70.

6. Berry SM, Connor JT, Lewis RJ. The platform trial: an efficient strategy for evaluating multiple treatments. *JAMA.* 2015;313(16):1619–20.

7. Angus DC, Alexander BM, Berry S, et al. Adaptive platform trials: definition, design, conduct and reporting considerations. *Nat Rev Drug Discov.* 2019;18(10):797–807.

8. Park JJH, Detry MA, Murthy S, Guyatt G, Mills EJ. How to use and interpret the results of a platform trial: users' guide to the medical literature. *JAMA.* 2022;327 (1):67–74.

9. Thorlund K, Dron L, Park J, Hsu G, Forrest JI, Mills EJ. A real-time dashboard of clinical trials for COVID-19. *Lancet Digit Health.* 2020;2(6):e286–e7.

10. Kanters S, Mills EJ, Thorlund K, Bucher HC, Ioannidis JP. Antiretroviral therapy for initial human immunodeficiency virus/AIDS treatment: critical appraisal of the evidence from over 100 randomized trials and 400 systematic reviews and meta-analyses. *Clin Microbiol Infect.* 2014;20(2):114–22.

11. Parmar MK, Carpenter J, Sydes MR. More multiarm randomised trials of superiority are needed. *Lancet.* 2014;384(9940):283–4.

12. Ventz S, Alexander BM, Parmigiani G, Gelber RD, Trippa L. Designing clinical trials that accept new arms: an example in metastatic breast cancer. *J Clin Oncolo.* 2017;35(27):3160–8.

13. Parmar MK, Barthel FM, Sydes M, et al. Speeding up the evaluation of new agents in cancer. *J Natl Cancer Inst.* 2008;100 (17):1204–14.

14. Sydes MR, Parmar MKB, James ND, et al. Issues in applying multi-arm multi-stage methodology to a clinical trial in prostate cancer: the MRC STAMPEDE trial. *Trials.* 2009;10:39.

15. Parmar MK, Sydes MR, Cafferty FH, et al. Testing many treatments within a single protocol over 10 years at MRC Clinical Trials Unit at UCL: multi-arm, multi-stage platform, umbrella and basket protocols. *Clin Trials.* 2017;14(5):451–61.

16. Mills EJ, Thorlund K, Ioannidis JP. Demystifying trial networks and network meta-analysis. *BMJ*. 2013;**346**:f2914.

17. Park JJH, Harari O, Dron L, et al. An overview of platform trials with a checklist for clinical readers. *J Clin Epidemiol*. 2020;**125**:1–8.

18. Angus DC, Derde L, Al-Beidh F, et al. Effect of hydrocortisone on mortality and organ support in patients with severe COVID-19: the REMAP-CAP COVID-19 Corticosteroid Domain Randomized Clinical Trial. *JAMA*. 2020;**324**(13):1317–29.

19. Recovery Collaborative Group, Horby P, Lim WS, Emberson JR, et al. Dexamethasone in hospitalized patients with Covid-19. *N Engl J Med*. 2021;**384**(8):693–704.

20. Park JJH, Mogg R, Smith GE, et al. How COVID-19 has fundamentally changed clinical research in global health. *Lancet Glob Health*. 2021;**9**(5):e711–e20.

21. Bugin K, Woodcock J. Trends in COVID-19 therapeutic clinical trials. *Nat Rev Drug Discov*. 2021;**20**(4):254–5.

22. Recovery Collaborative Group, Horby P, Lim WS, Emberson JR, et al. Dexamethasone in hospitalized patients with Covid-19 – preliminary report. *N Engl J Med*. 2020;**384**(8):693–704.

23. Beigel JH, Tomashek KM, Dodd LE, et al. Remdesivir for the treatment of Covid-19 – final report. *N Engl J Med*. 2020;**383**:1813–26.

24. Writing Committee for the Remap-CAP Investigators, Angus DC, Derde L, Al-Beidh F, et al. Effect of hydrocortisone on mortality and organ support in patients with severe COVID-19: the REMAP-CAP COVID-19 Corticosteroid Domain Randomized Clinical Trial. *JAMA*. 2020;**324**(13):1317–29.

25. Angus DC, Berry S, Lewis RJ, et al. The Randomized Embedded Multifactorial Adaptive Platform for Community-acquired Pneumonia (REMAP-CAP) study: rationale and design. *Ann Am Thorac Soc*. 2020;**17**(7):879–91.

26. Reis G, Moreira Silva E, Medeiros Silva DC, et al. Effect of early treatment with hydroxychloroquine or lopinavir and ritonavir on risk of hospitalization among patients with COVID-19: the TOGETHER Randomized Clinical Trial. *JAMA Netw Open*. 2021;**4**(4):e216468.

27. Group PTC. Azithromycin for community treatment of suspected COVID-19 in people at increased risk of an adverse clinical course in the UK (PRINCIPLE): a randomised, controlled, open-label, adaptive platform trial. *Lancet*. 2021;**397**(10279):1063–74.

28. Park JJH, Dron L, Mills EJ. Moving forward in clinical research with master protocols. *Contemp Clin Trials*. 2021;**106**:106438.

29. Saville BR, Berry SM. Efficiencies of platform clinical trials: a vision of the future. *Clin Trials*. 2016;**13**(3):358–66.

30. Adaptive Platform Trials C. Adaptive platform trials: definition, design, conduct and reporting considerations. *Nat Rev Drug Discov*. 2019;**18**(10):797–807.

31. Hummel J, Wang S, Kirkpatrick J. Using simulation to optimize adaptive trial designs: applications in learning and confirmatory phase trials. *Clin Invest*. 2015;**5**(4):401–13.

32. Viele K, McGlothlin A, Broglio K. Interpretation of clinical trials that stopped early. *Jama*. 2016;**315**(15):1646–7.

33. Park JJ, Thorlund K, Mills EJ. Critical concepts in adaptive clinical trials. *Clin Epidemiol*. 2018;**10**:343–51.

34. Biswas A, Bhattacharya R. Response-adaptive designs for continuous treatment responses in phase III clinical trials: a review. *Stat Methods Med Res*. 2016;**25**(1):81–100.

35. U.S. Department of Health and Human Services, Food and Drug Administration. *Adaptive Designs for Clinical Trials of Drugs and Biologics Guidance for Industry*. U.S. Department of Health and Human Services; 2019.

36. Thorlund K, Haggstrom J, Park JJ, Mills EJ. Key design considerations for adaptive clinical trials: a primer for clinicians. *BMJ*. 2018;**360**:k698.

37. Park JJH, Hsu G, Siden EG, Thorlund K, Mills EJ. An overview of precision oncology basket and umbrella trials for clinicians. *CA Cancer J Clin.* 2020;**70**(2):125–37.

38. Little RJ, Lewis RJ. Estimands, estimators, and estimates. *JAMA.* 2021;**326**(10):967–8.

39. Collignon O, Schiel A, Burman CF, et al. Estimands and complex innovative designs. *Clin Pharmacol Ther.* 2022. Online ahead of print.

40. Prentice RL. Surrogate endpoints in clinical trials: definition and operational criteria. *Stat Med.* 1989;**8**(4):431–40.

41. Haslam A, Hey SP, Gill J, Prasad V. A systematic review of trial-level meta-analyses measuring the strength of association between surrogate end-points and overall survival in oncology. *Eur J Cancer.* 2019;**106**:196–211.

42. Prasad V, Kim C, Burotto M, Vandross A. The strength of association between surrogate end points and survival in oncology: a systematic review of trial-level meta-analyses. *JAMA Intern Med.* 2015;**175**(8):1389–98.

43. Beauchemin C, Johnston JB, Lapierre ME, Aissa F, Lachaine J. Relationship between progression-free survival and overall survival in chronic lymphocytic leukemia: a literature-based analysis. *Curr Oncol (Toronto, Ont).* 2015;**22**(3):e148–56.

44. Cortazar P, Zhang JJ, Sridhara R, Justice RL, Pazdur R. Relationship between OS and PFS in metastatic breast cancer (MBC): review of FDA submission data. *J Clin Oncol.* 2011;**29**(15_suppl):1035.

45. Gyawali B, Hey SP, Kesselheim AS. A Comparison of response patterns for progression-free survival and overall survival following treatment for cancer with PD-1 inhibitors: a meta-analysis of correlation and differences in effect sizes. *JAMA Netw Open.* 2018;**1**(2):e180416–e.

46. Berry DA. Bayesian clinical trials. *Nat Rev Drug Discov.* 2006;**5**(1):27–36.

47. Saville BR, Connor JT, Ayers GD, Alvarez J. The utility of Bayesian predictive probabilities for interim monitoring of clinical trials. *Clin Trials.* 2014;**11**(4):485–93.

48. Lachin JM. A review of methods for futility stopping based on conditional power. *Stat Med.* 2005;**24**(18):2747–64.

49. Thorlund K, Golchi S, Haggstrom J, Mills E. Highly Efficient Clinical Trials Simulator (HECT): software application for planning and simulating platform adaptive trials. *Gates Open Res.* 2019;**3**:780.

50. Thorlund K, Golchi S, Mills E. Bayesian adaptive clinical trials of combination treatments. *Contemp Clin Trials Commun.* 2017;**8**:227–33.

51. Schiavone F, Bathia R, Letchemanan K, et al. This is a platform alteration: a trial management perspective on the operational aspects of adaptive and platform and umbrella protocols. *Trials.* 2019;**20**(1):264.

52. Hague D, Townsend S, Masters L, et al. Changing platforms without stopping the train: experiences of data management and data management systems when adapting platform protocols by adding and closing comparisons. *Trials.* 2019;**20**(1):294.

53. Dunnett CW. A multiple comparison procedure for comparing several treatments with a control. *JASA.* 1955;**50**(272):1096–121.

54. Berry SM, Petzold EA, Dull P, et al. A response adaptive randomization platform trial for efficient evaluation of Ebola virus treatments: a model for pandemic response. *Clin Trials.* 2016;**13**(1):22–30.

55. Sydes MR, Parmar MKB, Mason MD, et al. Flexible trial design in practice – stopping arms for lack-of-benefit and adding research arms mid-trial in STAMPEDE: a multi-arm multi-stage randomized controlled trial. *Trials.* 2012;**13**:168.

56. Barker AD, Sigman CC, Kelloff GJ, et al. I-SPY 2: an adaptive breast cancer trial design in the setting of neoadjuvant chemotherapy. *Clin Pharmacol Ther.* 2009;**86**(1):97–100.

57. Committee for Proprietary Medicinal Products. *ICH Topic E 10: Choice of Control*

Group in Clinical Trials., p. 30. European Medicines Agency (EMEA); 2001;

58. Thorlund K, Dron L, Park JJH, Mills EJ. Synthetic and external controls in clinical trials – a primer for researchers. *Clin Epidemiol.* 2020;**12**:457–67.

59. Lee KM, Wason J. Including non-concurrent control patients in the analysis of platform trials: is it worth it? *BMC Med Res Methodol.* 2020;**20**(1):165.

60. Berry SM, Reese CS, Larkey PD. Bridging different eras in sports. *JASA* 1999;**94**(447):661–76.

61. Viele K, Berry S, Neuenschwander B, et al. Use of historical control data for assessing treatment effects in clinical trials. *Pharm Stat.* 2014;**13**(1):41–54.

62. Dron L, Golchi S, Hsu G, Thorlund K. Minimizing control group allocation in randomized trials using dynamic borrowing of external control data – an application to second line therapy for non-small cell lung cancer. *Contemp Clin Trials Commun.* 2019;**16**:100446.

63. Yu LM, Bafadhel M, Dorward J, et al. Inhaled budesonide for COVID-19 in people at high risk of complications in the community in the UK (PRINCIPLE): a randomised, controlled, open-label, adaptive platform trial. *Lancet.* 2021;**398**(10303):843–55.

Basket Trials and Umbrella Trials

8

Jay J. H. Park, Edward J. Mills, and J. Kyle Wathen

Key Points of This Chapter

This chapter discusses characteristics of basket and umbrella trials and their key design considerations. The key points of this chapter are:

- Basket trials refer to clinical trials conducted to test one or more targeted therapies on multiple diseases that share common molecular alterations or other predictive risk factors.
- Umbrella trials refer to clinical trials that test two or more targeted therapies for a single disease that is stratified into multiple groups.
- In addition to sample size and randomisation considerations that are important to all clinical trials, specific design considerations that are important for basket and umbrella trials include biological plausibility of targeted intervention(s), accuracy of biomarker assays, biospecimen collection procedures, and prevalence of targeted biomarkers.

Introduction

There has been increased emphasis on biomarker-guided trials with biomarkers becoming a more integral part of clinical trial research [1, 2]. There are many different forms of biomarker-guided trials, but these trials generally utilise biomarker information to identify a group of patients who are more likely to benefit from the assigned intervention [3, 4]. Intervention strategies that aim to specifically affect (target) diseases based on their genetic make-up or other predictive risk factors are commonly referred to as targeted therapies [6–9]. In the previous chapters, we have discussed the concept of adaptive enrichment designs that allow for potential modification of trial eligibility criteria to a narrower group of patients (e.g., biomarker-positive sub-population) who may be more likely to benefit from an assigned intervention [3, 4]. Notable methodological advancements that have been made towards biomarker-guided clinical trials including the development of basket trials and umbrella trials under the master protocol framework [10–18]. In this chapter, we discuss the key characteristics of basket trials and umbrella trials, and how they compare with each other, other types of biomarker-guided trials, and adaptive trial designs, with a particular focus on adaptive enrichment designs. We also discuss key design considerations that are important for basket and umbrella trials.

Basket Trials and Umbrella Trials

Basket trials refer to clinical trials that test one or more targeted therapies across multiple types of diseases that share common molecular alterations or other predictive risk factors [10–13].

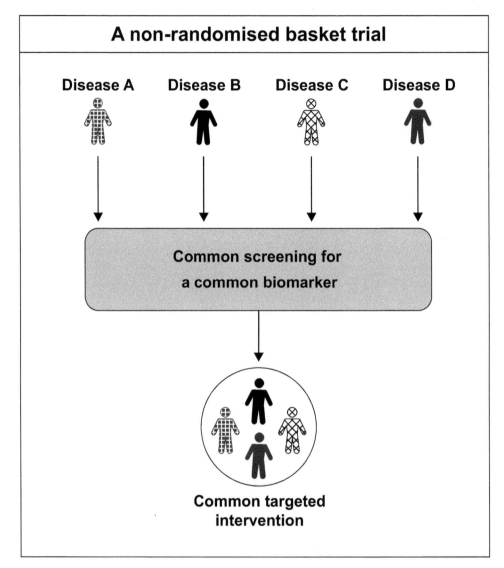

Figure 8.1 A single-arm non-randomised basket trial.

An illustrative example of a single-arm non-randomised basket trial without a control group is shown in this figure. Using a common screening, different diseases with a common biomarker target are recruited and assigned to a targeted intervention.

Basket trials have most commonly been applied in oncology and conducted as single-arm (non-randomised) trials (Figure 8.1), but it can be conducted as randomised clinical trials (Figure 8.2) [12]. In basket trials, there are unifying eligibility criteria that combine patients with different diseases into a single 'basket' or a single trial. The unifying eligibility criteria usually are based on a patient's predictive risk factor that is, in turn, based on the intervention's mechanism of action (or and specific molecular or other biomarkers as a target). Mechanism of action is often used as a target since it may help predict whether patients will respond to the assigned targeted therapy.

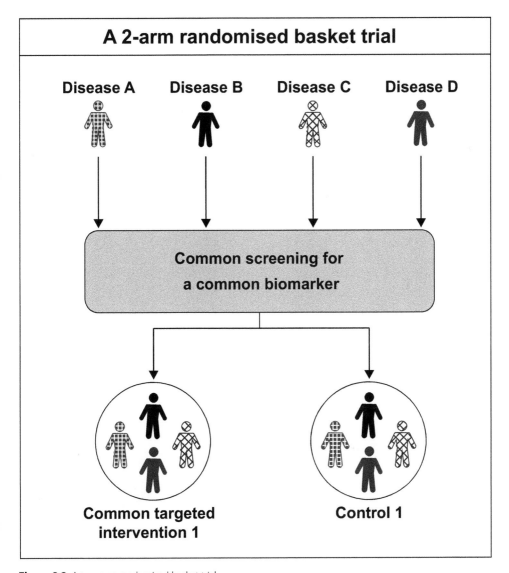

Figure 8.2 A two-arm randomised basket trial.

An illustrative example of a two-arm randomised basket trial with a control group is shown in this figure. Using a common screening, different diseases with a common biomarker target are recruited and randomly assigned to a targeted intervention arm or a control arm.

Umbrella trials, on the other hand, refer to clinical trials that test multiple (two or more) targeted interventions for a single disease based on predictive biomarkers or other predictive patient risk factors [10, 12, 13, 18, 19]. In umbrella trials, a single disease (e.g., advanced breast cancer) is stratified into multiple groups with each group's eligibility being defined by the intervention's mechanism of action or other molecular or other biomarkers. Similar to basket trials, umbrella trials have most commonly been applied in oncology and can be conducted with or without randomisation [12]. In contrast to basket trials, randomised

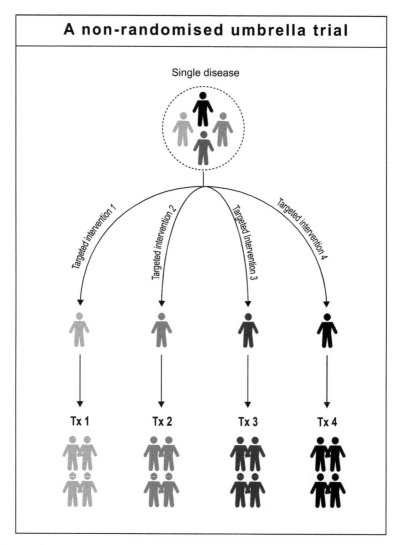

Figure 8.3 A multi-arm non-randomised umbrella trial.

An illustrative example of an umbrella trial using non-randomised design is shown here. Patients are assigned to a targeted therapy based on their eligibility criteria into one of four sub-studies in this umbrella trial. This target can be a biomarker or other predictive risk factor that may help predict their response to the assigned targeted therapy.

umbrella trials are more common than non-randomised trials [12]. An illustrative example of a non-randomised umbrella trial can be seen in Figure 8.3, and an example of a randomised umbrella trial can be seen in Figure 8.4.

Characteristics of Basket Trials and Umbrella Trials

Between basket and umbrella trials, there are important similarities and differences. Both designs aim to tailor intervention strategies based on the patient's risk factor(s) that can help predict whether they will respond to a specific treatment. They also use a master protocol to

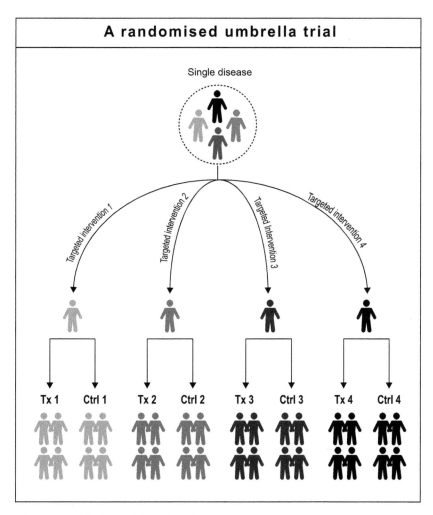

Figure 8.4 A multi-arm randomised umbrella trial.
An illustrative example of an umbrella trial using randomised design is shown here. Patients are assigned to one of four sub-studies based on their eligibility criteria. In each sub-study, they are randomly assigned to the respective targeted therapy or to the control group.

harmonise their clinical evaluation plan. For instance, in both basket and umbrella trials, a common screening protocol is employed to determine whether the patient is eligible. The majority of basket and umbrella trials conducted so far come from oncology and have been biomarker guided, so it is important to note that there was a common molecular screening protocol with standardised biomarker assays in these biomarker-guided trials [13]. In oncology, a basket trial would involve multiple histological types of cancer that share common biomarker targets for evaluation of one or more targeted therapies. Basket trials aim to identify tumour-agnostic therapies that can treat cancers based on their genetic and molecular alterations, regardless of their tumour types or where the cancer reside. Umbrella trials involve a single cancer type, such as lung cancer, but multiple biomarker targets and targeted interventions. Key differences between basket and umbrella trials exist in terms of their eligibility criteria, patient sub-grouping, and intervention assignment.

Eligibility Criteria and Patient Grouping

Patients enrolled in a basket trial will represent multiple diseases with a common unifying predictive risk factor, and in umbrella trials, patients with a common disease (a single disease) will be recruited and enrolled [13]. Umbrella trials have an inherent key methodological characteristic of using multiple predictive risk factors to determine patient sub-groups. Naturally, the use of patient sub-types is more common in these trials. In basket trials, patient sub-types may be defined based on their disease sub-types, given that the disease sub-type is often a prognostic factor; however, since multiple disease types of patients are recruited into a common cohort, 'unification of diseases' is a more appropriate way to describe the inherent nature of basket trials.

Patient grouping strategies are important to highlight since they are used to determine the types of patients who are recruited and how patients with different predictive risk factors are allocated to different interventions in basket and umbrella trials. While it is common for basket trials to have a targeted single intervention based on a common unifying predictive risk factor, it is possible for basket trials to have more than one targeted intervention. However, even in multi-arm basket trials, it is important to note that the clinical utilities of these interventions are usually assessed separately for each sub-study. Umbrella trials all have multiple targeted interventions (i.e., more than one intervention), and the clinical utilities of these interventions are usually assessed separately, with each sub-study being powered with its own assumptions and even sometimes having its own specific primary endpoints

Intervention Assignment and Choice in a Control Group

Both basket and umbrella trials may be conducted with or without control group (i.e., randomised vs. non-randomised designs). A landscape analysis conducted in 2019 showed that it is more common for umbrella trials to use a control group ($n = 8/18$, 44.4%) than basket trials ($n = 5/49$, 10.2%) [12]. For umbrella trials, the control group may be placebo if there is no established care, or the existing standard-of-care for the disease being studied may be used for all of the sub-types. Determining the control group can be more difficult in basket trials, since there are multiple diseases being studied. If there is no established care for all diseases being studied, the placebo may be used as the control group; if the diseases being studied in the basket trials have different standards-of-care, it may be possible that there may be different care being provided to the common control group. Of the four randomised basket trials that used a control group, two of them received no therapy (e.g., saline injection) or placebo [20, 21], and the control group in the other two basket trials received standards-of-care that were left to the discretion of the treating physician [22, 23].

Comparison against Other Biomarker-Guided Trials

Basket and umbrella trials share many similarities with other (non-master protocol) bio-marker-guided trials, but there are key differences that should be noted. In accordance with other biomarker-guided trials, the aim of basket and umbrella trial approaches is to utilise genomics and other '-omic' technologies to define disease and eligibility criteria for improved characterisation and identification of predictive biomarkers and targeted therapies. The use of a single master protocol with standardised operating procedures is a key difference from other types of non–master protocol biomarker-guided trials. Under the master protocol framework, basket and umbrella trials usually establish a large trial network and a common infrastructure across and through multiple institutions. Between these institutions, standardised operating procedures including a common screening mechanism are instituted for patient identification. Adopting a common molecular screening mechanism under a master protocol can help achieve screening efficiency for biomarker-guided trials.

In oncology-based basket trials, multiple cancers of different histopathologies are recruited into a single cohort when those cancers have common molecular alteration(s). Basket trials try to aim to identify histology-agnostic or tumour-agnostic therapies. Traditionally, it is not uncommon for phase I cancer clinical trials to recruit multiple types of histopathologies to test for the existence of signal, but basket trials and their histology-agnostic approaches are now being considered for phase II and even some phase III evaluations [12]. In umbrella trials, multiple histology-dependent targeted therapies are evaluated for multiple sub-groups of single histopathology that are molecularly differentiated through a common screening mechanism.

Screening for given biomarker(s) is an important consideration for biomarker-guided trials, as the number of patients required for the enrolment target will ultimately be dependent on the biomarker prevalence of interest. For instance, if the group of interest is breast cancer patients harbouring a specific mutation, the number of breast cancer patients who will need to be screened will depend on the biomarker prevalence of interest. If we assume that 10% of breast cancer patients will have the specific mutation of interest, it can be expected that roughly 2,000 patients will need to be screened to reach the recruitment target size of 200 patients. Umbrella trials can be conducted independently as multiple trials for each of the molecular targets of interest. However, it is important to note that conducting these trials independently would require a much larger number of patients who would need to be screened collectively.

Comparison against Adaptive Trial Designs

Basket trials and umbrella trials refer to specific types of clinical trials conducted to evaluate targeted therapies that are often guided by biomarkers. The targeted therapy strategy in basket trials involves unification of multiple diseases into a single 'basket', whereas umbrella trials combine evaluation of multiple targeted therapies under one common 'umbrella'. Neither basket nor umbrella trials, by definition, are adaptive clinical trials. They can be conducted with a fixed sample trial design, where one final analysis is conducted at the target sample size or number of events. Adaptive trial designs merely refer to clinical trial designs that specify how the trials will respond to the accumulating data. Adaptive trial designs can be used to improve flexibility in how basket and umbrella trials are conducted, but they are not interchangeable.

Comparison of basket and umbrella trials versus adaptive enrichment designs deserves further discussion. Comparable to basket and umbrella trials, clinical trials with adaptive enrichment designs are often biomarker guided and aim to identify targeted intervention strategies. Adaptive enrichment designs commonly involve a single disease and a single biomarker. Such a trial would usually start by enrolling an all-comers (e.g., biomarker positive and negative) population, but it would allow for potential adaptation to restrict further enrolment to the sub-population (e.g., biomarker-positive patients) that is more likely to benefit from the therapy being evaluated. To our knowledge, the basket and umbrella trials conducted thus far have no such possible enrichment designs, and they usually start with the targeted group(s) who are hypothesised to benefit from the interventions being studied [12].

Key Design Considerations for Basket Trials and Umbrella Trials

There are several key design considerations for basket and umbrella trials (Table 8.1). These include consideration of biological plausibility of the underlying targeted therapy strategies, accuracy of biomarker assays being adopted, biospecimen collection, and biomarker prevalence. As with any clinical trials, there are sample size considerations and potential risk of bias considerations when randomisation is not used.

Biological Plausibility

It is important to consider the biological plausibility of the targeted intervention strategies being evaluated. Basket and umbrella trial designs have both been developed under the core principle of precision medicine that aims to tailor medical intervention based on the patient's characteristics that make them more likely to respond to that intervention (i.e., predictive risk factors). The underlying biological plausibility assumption is therefore critical for these trials, since information on the diseases being studied and the treatment's mechanisms of actions will be used to derive targeted intervention strategies.

For instance, it is common for cancers to have multiple genetic mutations; however, it is important to note that only some of these may be 'driver mutations' for the carcinogenic process, with most mutations being 'passenger mutations' that do not affect the underlying carcinogenic process [24]. Intervention strategies should, of course, be targeting driver mutations, but it can be difficult to differentiate driver mutations from passenger mutations [24, 25]. Careful consideration of the pre-clinical evidence and underlying biological models informing the targeted intervention strategies will need to be made for critical appraisal of both basket and umbrella trials.

Accuracy of Biomarker Assays

In addition to biomarker plausibility, it is critical to consider the accuracy of biomarker assays that are used in basket and umbrella trials. Conceptually, a targeted intervention should be more efficacious against diseases demonstrating characteristics of the biomarker target versus diseases that do not possess the target. However, all medical tests will have some degree of diagnostic inaccuracy, and so a proportion of biomarker false negative and false positive patients are expected in biomarker-guided basket and umbrella trials. It has been shown that increasing false positive rates (FPRs) of biomarker tests will reduce the statistical power in early exploratory biomarker-guided trials; while it has not been a common practice, FPRs of biomarker tests should be incorporated in the planning of these biomarker-guided trials [26]. Careful considerations of the accuracy of biomarker assays are important for exploratory (i.e., phase II) basket and umbrella trials in order to improve the probability of selecting suitable candidates for further testing (i.e., phase III) [26]. For basket trials, it is important that the accuracies of biomarker assays are similar between different tumour types.

Table 8.1 Key considerations for basket and umbrella trials
Several key design considerations for basket and umbrella trials are summarised in this table.

Key considerations	Details
Biological plausibility	• Careful evaluations of the pre-existing clinical evidence and underlying biological assumptions are required to ensure that there is a biological plausibility for the targeted interventions.
Accuracy of biomarker tests	• Accuracy of biomarker tests is important, but since all medical tests will have some degree of inaccuracy, it is important to account for inaccuracy (i.e., false positive rates) in the trial planning stage to avoid underpowering the trial. • If there are multiple tumour types involved, the accuracy of biomarker tests should be similar between these tumours.
Biospecimen collection	• The biospecimen collection process should be easy, and relatively uniform high biospecimen quality and biospecimen yield must be achievable, especially for basket trials that have multiple diseases.
Biomarker prevalence	• Prevalence of biomarker(s) used should be anticipated with possible recruitment challenges.
Sample size and assumptions	• The sample size requirements for randomised basket and umbrella trials are generally larger than those trials with single-arm designs. • In basket and umbrella trials with single-arm designs without a control arm, the planned sample size should be sufficient to rule out clinically important treatment effects. • In randomised designs, sample size calculations may be done for the common cohort in basket trials or for each of the sub-groups in umbrella trials. • Recruitment may be more favourable for basket trials that can recruit from pools of patients of multiple diseases. Umbrella trials may be harder for recruitment since it can only be done from a sub-set of one patient disease pool.
Randomisation	• Targeted intervention strategies rely on predictive risk factors that determine whether the patient will respond to a given intervention. • Use of randomisation and a control group with adequate sample size can determine whether the risk factor is predictive or not. • If randomisation is not feasible, statistical adjustments can be made. However, there are issues with making statistical adjustments with smaller datasets. • If there is adequate sample size, it is important to note that statistical adjustments can only account for measurable factors.

Biospecimen Collection

Careful considerations for biospecimen collection procedures will be important, particularly for basket trials that involve multiple histological tumours. Ease of biospecimen collection, biospecimen quality, and biospecimen yield should be similar between different tumours. Outside of direct measures of test performance, appropriate biopsy yield can be challenging [27]. Even at high throughput centres with skilled technicians, a yield as low as

70% for adequate lung adenocarcinoma molecular profiling via biopsy has been reported [28]. Advances in sampling methodologies and techniques such as liquid biopsy [29] may represent less invasive ways to investigate molecular profiling, but their test performance must be carefully considered against their benefits to patient experience, and the importance of histopathological examination should not be underestimated [30].

Biomarker Prevalence

Patient recruitment is critical for any clinical trial [31]. Thus, it is important to consider the prevalence of biomarkers that will be used in both basket and umbrella trials since the biomarker prevalence will affect the size of the patient pool eligible for these biomarker-guided trials. A low biomarker prevalence would translate to a small pool of eligible patients, and a high prevalence would translate to a larger patient pool. If the biomarker prevalence is low for basket trials, there may be serious recruitment challenges in that it may not be feasible to recruit the planned sample size within the planned duration of the trial. Similarly, if the biomarker prevalence is low in one or more arms in umbrella trials, it will be difficult to recruit patients harbouring the specific mutation for that intervention arm(s). Planning for comprehensive recruitment strategies to reach the target sample size within the trial duration will therefore be especially vital for biomarker-guided basket and umbrella trials where the prevalence of biomarker-positive patients is low. Low biomarker prevalence will likely result in high screening failure, so financial cost considerations of obtaining biospecimens (e.g., biopsies) and running the biomarker testing are important.

Sample Sizes and Assumptions

As with all types of clinical trials, sample size considerations are important for basket and umbrella trials. The sample size for a given basket or umbrella trial will depend on its clinical phase. Sample size requirements for exploratory (phase II) trials are smaller than confirmatory (phase III) trials, since exploratory trials act as a screening tool to assess whether an intervention warrants further investigation [32]. In exploratory trials, single-arm designs without a control arm (non-randomised design, phase IIA) or randomised designs (phase IIB) may be used [26, 32]. For single-arm designs, the U.S. Food and Drug Administration (FDA) recommends that the planned sample size should be sufficient to rule out a clinically unimportant treatment effect in non-randomised designs, and it recommends designs such as the Simon's two-stage design in order to limit exposure to an ineffective intervention [11, 33].

For basket trials, sample size calculations may be done for the overall cohort that consists of multiple diseases. If this is the case, one treatment effect size will be used as an input for the sample size calculation. That is, the underlying assumption of the common predictive risk factor being used for the unification of diseases in a given basket trial must be valid. For instance, if the targeted therapy being studied in a multi-histology basket trial has different treatment effects between different tumours (e.g., the treatment only works well in one tumour), the clinical efficacy of the therapy may be underestimated since the overall treatment effect observed may be diluted due to non-responding tumours that were included in the trial. In basket trials that show non-promising results overall, it can be difficult to determine whether and which disease sub-type(s) may respond to the therapy being studied, since they are sub-groups.

The sample size calculations for umbrella trials, on the other hand, may be done for each of the sub-groups since there are multiple targeted interventions being evaluated in umbrella trials. If possible, the FDA has recommended the use of a common control arm for umbrella trials [11]. Regardless, the assumptions that the risk factors being used are predictive are also critical for umbrella trials. For example, if a given intervention is truly effective and the predictive risk factor assumption is erroneous, the clinical efficacy of the given targeted therapy will only be investigated in a sub-population instead of the general population (e.g., all-comers). Therefore, an all-comers design strategy instead of the enrichment trial design strategy used in umbrella trials may be better if the predictive risk factor assumption is erroneous, since the all-comers strategy would have found the intervention to be effective for the entire general disease population.

If the predictive risk factor assumption is valid (or reasonable), the basket and umbrella trial designs would be more favourable than the all-comers designs. The sample size requirements for a given treatment effect size will be similar between the enrichment and all-comers design approaches. However, recruitment will be more favourable for basket trials that can recruit from pools of patients with multiple diseases; conversely, it may be difficult to recruit patients for umbrella trials given that recruitment can only be done from a subset of one patient disease pool.

Randomisation

Predictive risk factors refer to patient characteristics that are associated with their response (or lack of response) to a particular intervention [34, 35]. Predictive risk factors are used in both basket and umbrella trials to inform their targeted intervention strategies. Prognostic factors, on the other hand, refer to patient characteristics that affect the clinical outcome independent of the intervention [34, 35]. The patient's clinical outcome is determined by their prognostic risk factors, regardless of whether they were treated or not, so it is important to distinguish between predictive and prognostic risk factors when assessing intervention utility. However, in basket and umbrella trials that do not use randomisation, it may be difficult to determine whether the biomarker used for a given intervention strategy is a predictive factor or a prognostic factor.

Randomisation removes selection bias and tends to produce groups that are comparable in terms of both measurable and unmeasurable factors [36]. Randomisation therefore helps to ascribe the observed difference in the treatment effects to the interventions that are being compared in a given trial, allowing for the establishment of causality [36, 37]. In single-arm basket and umbrella trials, it can be difficult to differentiate between predictive and prognostic factors. For instance, the clinical efficacy of a given experimental intervention may be overestimated in single-arm basket trials with a unifying risk factor that has a favourable prognosis. Similarly, in umbrella trials, the sub-group arm(s) with a favourable prognostic risk factor may result in overestimated treatment effects. On the other hand, if an unfavourable prognostic risk factor is used as the predictive intervention strategy, the treatment effects may be underestimated in both basket and umbrella trials. In these trials, randomisation can help determine whether the risk factors being used as part of the targeted intervention strategies are indeed predictive, since randomisation can help achieve a balance of measurable and unmeasurable prognostic factors between the experimental and control groups.

If randomisation is not feasible, it may be possible to make statistical adjustments to ameliorate potential biases and imbalances to differentiate predictive risk factors versus prognostic risk factors. However, statistical adjustments are difficult in smaller datasets, and so even an adjusted analyses cannot lead to unbiased estimates, if the sample size is small [38]. Even if there is adequate sample size, it is important to note that statistical adjustments can only account for measurable factors. Thus, the use of randomisation is generally preferable.

Conclusion

In this chapter, we have discussed key characteristics of basket and umbrella trials as well as several important considerations that need to be made for these clinical trials in terms of biological plausibility, biomarker test accuracy and prevalence, sample sizes, and predictive or prognostic significance of the biomarker used for the targeted intervention strategies. As basket and umbrella trials inherently share similarities with other biomarker-guided trials, the design considerations reviewed in this chapter likely apply to other biomarker-guided trials as well. The framework of master protocols that aim to establish a common screening mechanism with standardised operating procedures is a key difference of basket and umbrella trials from other biomarker-guided trials.

References

1. Heckman-Stoddard BM, Smith JJ. Precision medicine clinical trials: defining new treatment strategies. *Semin Oncol Nurs.* 2014;30(2):109–16.

2. Berry DA. The brave new world of clinical cancer research: adaptive biomarker-driven trials integrating clinical practice with clinical research. *Mol Oncol.* 2015;9 (5):951–9.

3. Antoniou M, Jorgensen AL, Kolamunnage-Dona R. Biomarker-guided adaptive trial designs in phase II and phase III: a methodological review. *PloS ONE.* 2016;11 (2):e0149803.

4. Antoniou M, Kolamunnage-Dona R, Jorgensen AL. Biomarker-guided non-adaptive trial designs in phase II and phase III: a methodological review. *J Pers Med.* 2017;7(1).

5. Kumar-Sinha C, Chinnaiyan AM. Precision oncology in the age of integrative genomics. *Nat Biotechnol.* 2018;36(1):46–60.

6. Abrams J, Conley B, Mooney M, et al. National Cancer Institute's Precision Medicine Initiatives for the new National Clinical Trials Network. *Am Soc Clin Oncol Educ Book.* 2014:71–6.

7. Collins FS, Varmus H. A new initiative on precision medicine. *N Engl J Med.* 2015;372 (9):793–5.

8. Ashley EA. The precision medicine initiative: a new national effort. *JAMA.* 2015;313(21):2119–20.

9. Ashley EA. Towards precision medicine. *Nat Rev Genet.* 2016;17(9):507–22.

10. Woodcock J, LaVange LM. Master protocols to study multiple therapies, multiple diseases, or both. *N Eng J Med* 2017;377(1):62–70.

11. U.S. Department of Health and Human Services, Food and Drug Administration. Master Protocols: Efficient Clinical Trial Design Strategies to Expedite Development of Oncology Drugs and Biologics Guidance for Industry (Draft Guidance). U.S. Department of Health and Human Services; 2018. www.fda .gov/downloads/Drugs/Guidance ComplianceRegulatoryInformation/ Guidances/UCM621817.pdf.

12. Park JJH, Siden E, Zoratti MJ, et al. Systematic review of basket trials, umbrella trials, and platform trials: a landscape analysis of master protocols. *Trials.* 2019;20(1):572.

13. Siden EG, Park JJ, Zoratti MJ, et al. Reporting of master protocols towards a standardized approach: a systematic review. *Contemp Clin Trials Commun.* 2019;15:100406.

14. Hirakawa A, Asano J, Sato H, Teramukai S. Master protocol trials in oncology: review and new trial designs. *Contemp Clin Trials Commun.* 2018;**12**:1–8.

15. Lam VK, Papadimitrakopoulou V. Master protocols in lung cancer: experience from Lung Master Protocol. *Curr Opin Oncol.* 2018;**30**(2):92–7.

16. Ledford H. 'Master protocol' aims to revamp cancer trials: pilot project will bring drug companies together to test targeted lung-cancer therapies. *Nature.* 2013;**498**(7453):146–8.

17. Redman MW, Allegra CJ. The master protocol concept. *Semin Oncol.* 2015;**42** (5):724–30.

18. Renfro LA, Sargent DJ. Statistical controversies in clinical research: basket trials, umbrella trials, and other master protocols: a review and examples. *Ann Oncol.* 2017;**28**(1):34–43.

19. Parmar MK, Sydes MR, Cafferty FH, et al. Testing many treatments within a single protocol over 10 years at MRC Clinical Trials Unit at UCL: multi-arm, multi-stage platform, umbrella and basket protocols. *Clin Trials.* 2017;**14**(5):451–61.

20. De Benedetti F, Gattorno M, Anton J, et al. Canakinumab for the treatment of autoinflammatory recurrent fever syndromes. *N Engl J Med.* 2018;**378** (20):1908–19.

21. Muhlbacher J, Jilma B, Wahrmann M, et al. Blockade of HLA antibody-triggered classical complement activation in sera from subjects dosed with the anti-C1s monoclonal antibody TNT009 – results from a randomized first-in-human phase 1 trial. *Transplantation.* 2017;**101** (10):2410–18.

22. The ASCO Post. 2018 ASCO: IMPACT Trial matches treatment to genetic changes in the tumor to improve survival across multiple cancer types. 2018. www.ascopost.com/News/58897

23. Le Tourneau C, Delord JP, Goncalves A, et al. Molecularly targeted therapy based on tumour molecular profiling versus conventional therapy for advanced cancer

24. (SHIVA): a multicentre, open-label, proof-of-concept, randomised, controlled phase 2 trial. *Lancet Oncol.* 2015;**16** (13):1324–34.

24. Pon JR, Marra MA. Driver and passenger mutations in cancer. *Annu Rev Pathol.* 2015;**10**:25–50.

25. Brown AL, Li M, Goncearenco A, Panchenko AR. Finding driver mutations in cancer: elucidating the role of background mutational processes. *PLoS Comput Biol.* 2019;**15**(4):e1006981.

26. Park JJ, Harari O, Dron L, Mills EJ, Thorlund K. Effects of biomarker diagnostic accuracy on biomarker-guided phase 2 trials. *Contemp Clin Trials Commun.* 2019;**15**:100396.

27. Bubendorf L, Lantuejoul S, de Langen AJ, Thunnissen E. Nonsmall cell lung carcinoma: diagnostic difficulties in small biopsies and cytological specimens: number 2 in the series 'Pathology for the Clinician' edited by Peter Dorfmuller and Alberto Cavazza. *Eur Respir Rev.* 2017;**26**(144).

28. Iding JS, Krimsky W, Browning R. Tissue requirements in lung cancer diagnosis for tumor heterogeneity, mutational analysis and targeted therapies: initial experience with intra-operative Frozen Section Evaluation (FROSE) in bronchoscopic biopsies. *J Thorac Dis.* 2016;**8**(Suppl 6): S488–S93.

29. Arneth B. Update on the types and usage of liquid biopsies in the clinical setting: a systematic review. *BMC Cancer.* 2018 Dec;**18**(1):1–2.

30. Heitzer E, Ulz P, Geigl JB. Circulating tumor DNA as a liquid biopsy for cancer. *Clin Chem.* 2015;**61**(1):112–23.

31. Huang GD, Bull J, Johnston McKee K, et al. Clinical trials recruitment planning: a proposed framework from the Clinical Trials Transformation Initiative. *Contemp Clin Trials.* 2018;**66**:74–9.

32. Brown SR, Gregory WM, Twelves CJ, et al. Designing phase II trials in cancer: a systematic review and guidance. *Br J Cancer.* 2011;**105**(2):194–9.

33. Simon R. Optimal two-stage designs for phase II clinical trials. *Control Clin Trials.* 1989;**10**(1):1–10.

34. Clark GM, Zborowski DM, Culbertson JL, et al. Clinical utility of epidermal growth factor receptor expression for selecting patients with advanced non-small cell lung cancer for treatment with erlotinib. *J Thorac Oncol.* 2006;**1**(8):837–46.

35. Clark GM. Prognostic factors versus predictive factors: examples from a clinical trial of erlotinib. *Mol Oncol.* 2008;**1**(4):406–12.

36. Friedman LM, Furberg C, DeMets DL, Reboussin D, Granger CB. *Fundamentals of Clinical Trials*: Springer; 2015.

37. Cartwright N. What are randomised controlled trials good for? *Phil Stud.* 2010;**147**(1):59.

38. Roberts C, Torgerson DJ. Understanding controlled trials: baseline imbalance in randomised controlled trials. *BMJ.* 1999;**319**(7203):185.

Case Studies of Adaptive Trial Designs

9

Jay J. H. Park, Edward J. Mills, and J. Kyle Wathen

Introduction

This chapter is intended to complement the previous chapters by providing a collection of case studies of adaptive trial designs across various disciplines. We have organised the case studies by their main adaptive design feature. Each case study describes the background of individual trial and summarises key design details and overall results. Our presentation and discussion do not necessarily represent the official view of the trial investigators. Our discussion is intended to improve the reader's general literacy and comprehension of published results of adaptive clinical trials.

Group Sequential Design

Case Study 9.1: MUSEC Trial (NCT00552604)

Background

MUltiple Sclerosis and Extract of Cannabis (MUSEC) was a phase III, placebo-controlled, double-blinded, randomised trial evaluating an oral cannabis extract as a treatment for muscle stiffness in patients with stable multiple sclerosis (NCT00552604) [1]. As a result of increased tone and spasms, muscle stiffness can frequently occur in MS patients, leadiing to considerable distress, pain, reduced mobility, and overall compromised quality of life [2]. The trial investigators conducted MUSEC to test their hypothesis about oral cannabis extract supplying symptomatic relief of muscle stiffness and pain in adults (18–64 years old) with MS [1]. MUSEC is a case study of a group sequential design.

Design and Methods

Adult MS patients who had stable disease for the past 6 months and trouble with muscle stiffness for at least 3 months were randomly assigned to the cannabis or to the placebo arm at a 1:1 allocation ratio [1]. Patients had undergone a 2-week dose titration phase followed by a 10-week maintenance phase, with follow-up schedule of 2, 4, 8, and 12 weeks. The patient rating of their muscle stiffness relief was measured on an 11-point scale (0 indicated 'very much better', 5 indicated 'no difference', and 10 indicated 'very much worse') that asked patients to rate their stiffness over the last week compared to what it had been prior to the study [1]. The ratings in the range of 0 to 3 were deemed as a clinically relevant response and used to classify the response as having muscle stiffness relief. The primary endpoint was a rate of muscle stiffness relief (0 to 3 vs. 4 to 11) assessed at 12 weeks.

Comparison of the rate of the reported muscle stiffness relief at 12 weeks between the treatment and the placebo groups based on an intention-to-treat (as randomised) principle was defined as the primary analysis for this trial. The maximum sample size of 400 patients per arm was determined based on assumptions of a 27% response rate in the placebo group and a targeted treatment effect of 15% absolute increase for an overall response rate of 42%.

Under these assumptions, recruiting 340 evaluable participants (170 per group) would allow for 80% power with one-sided type I error rate of 0.025, but a 15% dropout rate was expected, so the target enrolment was set at 400 patients (200 per group). MUSEC planned for a single interim analysis that would allow for early stopping based on superiority [1]. An interim analysis was planned at the sample size of 200 (information fraction of 0.50) using the O'Brien–Fleming stopping boundary that set the stopping boundary at an alpha of 0.0026 [1, 3]. Based on the interim analysis, the independent Data and Safety Monitoring Board (DSMB) had recommended a change in the overall sample size target from 400 to 300 on the basis that it would be enough to maintain a conditional power of 95% [1]. The significance level for the final analysis was planned at 0.024 to preserve an overall type I error rate control at 0.025.

Findings

The MUSEC reports their findings based on the final analysis that included 279 patients (144 to treatment and 135 to placebo), who were randomised between June 2006 and September 2008 [1]. The response rate observed was 29.4% in the treatment group and 15.7% in the placebo group. While the response rates in both groups were lower than planned rates, the observed rates translated to an odds ratio of 2.26 (95% CI: 1.24, 4.13) with a p-value (one-sided) of 0.004. As the observed p-value was lower than the final significance level (0.004 < 0.024), the cannabis extract was concluded as being superior for treating muscle stiffness among MS adult patients.

While MUSEC is a relatively straightforward case example of a sequential design that had been able to complete the trial at a reduced sample size than originally planned, there are some concerns in reporting. There are no details presented in the use of conditional power for sample size re-assessment, and it does not appear to be a formal rule that was pre-specified ahead of time. It is not uncommon for the DSMB to recommend changes to the design that are not planned. Recall from our discussion in Chapter 4 that group sequential tests such as the O'Brien–Fleming stopping boundary require equal spacing between scheduled analyses. This trial planned for one interim analysis at 200 patients (information fraction of 0.50) and a final analysis at 400 patients, but the final analysis was based on 279 patients, at an information fraction of 0.6975, of the originally planned sample size [1]. While this perhaps may be a trivial discussion, it is important to maintain transparency and provide adequate reporting of adaptive trial designs [4, 5].

Case Study 9.2: Vitamin C, Thiamine, and Steroids in Sepsis (VICTAS; NCT03509350)

Background

Vitamin C, Thiamine, and Steroids in Sepsis (VICTAS) is a double-blinded, placebo-controlled, adaptive randomised clinical trial with sequential design conducted to evaluate the combined use of vitamin C, thiamine, and corticosteroids as a potential therapeutic option for critically ill patients with sepsis (NCT03509350) [6–8]. This trial was conducted to demonstrate the efficacy of this combination therapy versus matching placebos for organ functions and mortality in sepsis patients. VICTAS was designed to have flexible sample size with multiple sequential stopping rules with multiple end-points based on predictive probabilities [7].

Design and Methods

The target population of VICTAS included adult patients (18 or older) with acute respiratory and/or cardiovascular dysfunction with suspected infection of sepsis admit-ted to the intensive care unit (ICU) [6]. Patients were randomised in a 1:1 ratio to the intervention or the control group using permuted block randomisation with varying blocks (2, 4, or 6) that was stratified at each site. The primary endpoint was the number of ventilator- and vasopressor-free days in the first 30 days following randomisation, with mortality within 30 days of randomisation as a key secondary endpoint. The trial was designed to detect 1.5 ventilatory- and vasopressor-free days with the maximum recruitment of 2,000 patients [7].

Interim analyses where recruitment could be stopped earlier than 2,000 were planned when 200, 300, 400, 500, 1,000, and 1,500 patients were randomised between the treatment and control groups [7]. During the first 400 patients being enrolled, the interim analyses for early superiority stopping were permitted based on the mortality endpoint on the basis that the trial will stop recruitment for the evidence of an overwhelming benefit on the mortality endpoint. The trial planned to continue onto the larger sample size if no conclusive benefit to mortality could be detected. Beyond 400 patients, it was designed that both interim and final analyses would be based on the ventilatory- and vasopressor-free days as the primary endpoint with mortality as a key secondary endpoint.

Decision rules used for VICTAS are summarised in Table 9.1. Each interim analysis used day 30 observations that were monitored or imputed if not yet available. For early interim analyses on mortality (200, 300, and 400 patients), the trial could be stopped early for superiority if the predictive probability of success on the mortality endpoint was higher than 90%. The predictive probability of success on mortality refers to the probability of eventual success at the current sample size when all currently enrolled subjects finished their 30-day follow-up. For the calculation of predictive probability on mortality, an eventual success was defined by achieving significance on mortality with a one-sided alpha of 0.001.

For interim analyses that were planned beyond the sample size of 400 patients (500, 1,000, and 1,500 patients), the trial could stop early based on superiority or futility. There were two stopping rules for superiority and one stopping rule for futility. Early superiority stopping could be allowed based on both endpoints or ventilatory- and vasopressor-free days endpoint alone. The trial could stop early if the predictive probability of eventual success at the current sample size exceeded 95% for both endpoints, or based on ventilatory- and vasopressor-free days endpoint only, if its predictive probability of superiority for this endpoint at the current sample size was greater than 95%, but the predictive probability for mortality at the maximum sample size was less than 10%. The trial could be stopped early for futility when there were less than 10% predictive probabilities of superiority for ventilatory- and vasopressor-free days at the maximum sample size. In the calculation of these predictive probabilities, an eventual success was defined as achieving significance at a one-sided alpha of 0.022%.

In a complex trial such as VICTAS that utilises multiple stopping rules, there are no closed-form expressions (mathematical equations that use a finite number of operations), so trial simulations are required to assess the operating characteristics. As it was required, the decision rules at each interim analysis of VICTAS were calibrated using trial simulations (simulation size of 1,000 times) to control the one-sided type I error rate at 0.025 and estimate

Table 9.1 Decision rules for interim analyses in VICTAS [7]

Endpoint	Decision rule for superiority	Decision rule for futility
Interim analyses at sample size of 200, 300, and 400[*]		
30-day mortality	Predictive probability of superiority at current sample size for mortality > 90%	–
Interim analyses at sample size of 500, 1,000, and 1,500[**]		
Both endpoints	Predictive probability of superiority at current sample size > 95% in both endpoints	–
Ventilatory- and vasopressor-free days (VVFD) only	Predictive probability of superiority at current sample size for VVFD > 95% & predictive probability of superiority at maximum sample size for mortality < 10%	Predictive probability of superiority at maximum sample size for VVFD < 10%

[*] For interim analyses at sample size <500, an eventual success was defined by achieving significance on mortality with one-sided alpha of 0.001.
[**] For interim analyses at sample size of 500 or greater, an eventual success was defined by achieving significance at one-sided alpha of 0.022.

the statistical power. The expected statistical power varied between different assumptions about treatment effects. When a mortality benefit of 20% was assumed, the expected power of 99% to detect a mortality benefit could be expected, with the trial stopping early at or before a sample size of 500 patients [6, 7].

Findings

The results of VICTAS were published in the *Journal of the American Medical Association* (*JAMA*) on 23 February 2021 [6]. The VICTAS reports their results based on a total of 501 patients (252 to the intervention group and 249 to the control group) who were enrolled between August 2018 and July 2019 [6]. The median ventilator- and vasopressor-free days were 25 days (interquartile range [IQR]: 0, 29 days) for the intervention group and 26 days (IQR: 0, 28 days) for the placebo group with a median difference of –1 day (95% CI: –4, 2 days). The 30-day mortality rates were 22% in the intervention group and 24% in the placebo groups. There were no important differences observed in either the ventilatory- and vasopressor-free days or mortality endpoints.

VICTAS did not stop early based on the pre-specified rules that the investigators had planned for, but rather the trial was terminated early based on an administrative reason. According to the authors, the funder actually withheld additional funding that could allow for completion of the trial due to a change in their priorities [6]. This trial is controversial for another reason. The editors of *JAMA* made a statement about their concern over the lack of DSMB membership in the VICTAS trial [9]. It was reported that an individual who served as the chair of the DSMB was also involved in the initial trial design and in the statistical analysis and interpretation of the data [9]. The DSMB was not involved in the decision that led to early termination and withdrew support, so concerns in this specific instance might be minimal. However, independent functioning of the DSMB members is required, especially in complex adaptive clinical trials, to help ensure scientific standards, safety, and integrity of the trial conduct.

Seamless Design

Case Study 9.3: Broad-Spectrum HPV Vaccine Study (NCT00543543)

Background

Human papillomavirus (HPV) infection causes nearly all cervical cancers [10, 11]. HPV-16 and HPV-18 are two types of HPV that are known to cause about 70% of HPV-related cervical cancers [10, 11]. At the time of this case study, 4-valent HPV vaccine that addresses four HPV types (6, 11, 16, and 18) has been the gold standard for HPV vaccines [12]. As 4-valent HPV vaccine covers HPV-16 and HPV-18, they are believed to provide approximately 70% protection of cervical cancers. The investigators of this case study hypothesised that an HPV vaccine, such as 9-valent HPV that covers a broader spectrum of HPVs, could potentially offer an increased protection for cervical cancers [13]. To test this hypothesis, they conducted a seamless phase IIB/III trial to evaluate the efficacy and safety of 9-valent HPV vaccine versus the gold standard in 4-valent HPV vaccine as a control (NCT00543543) [13, 14].

Design and Methods

This trial started as a phase IIB trial with three different formulations with varying doses (low, medium, and high) of 9-valent HPV vaccine with the goal of identifying an optimal formulation for the phase III evaluation (Table 9.2) [13]. The three formulations of 9-valent were three-dose regimens with two subsequent doses being administered at month 2 and month 6 after the first dose, but with varying concentrations that could be characterised as 'low-dose', 'medium-dose', and 'high-dose' [13]. The control group with 4-valent HPV followed the same dosing schedule.

Table 9.2 Overview of trial design for NCT00543543

Intervention group	Control group	Target sample size or events	Primary analysis[*]
		Phase IIB	
Three doses of 9-valent HPV vaccine: Low/ medium/high	4-valent HPV vaccine	1,240 (310 per arm)	Non-inferiority testing of antibody response
		Phase III	
One dose of 9-valent HPV vaccine selected from phase IIB	4-valent HPV vaccine	30 events and 14,000 patients (7,000 per arm)	Superiority testing of high-grade cervical, vulvar, or vaginal disease related to HPV-31, -33, -45, -52, and -58 (strains covered by 9-valent HPV vaccine and not by 4-valent HPV vaccine).

[*] Per-protocol analysis group, defined by those who received three full doses and provided their 7-month serum sample, was used for the primary analyses of both phases IIB and III.

The enrolment target for phase IIB portion of this trial was set at 310 patients per group (a total of 1,240 subjects) to obtain 209 to 230 evaluable patients per arm assuming an attrition rate of 10% [13]. This was determined with the primary analysis being defined based on per-protocol analysis of non-inferiority of antibody responses to four types of HPVs that are protected by the control group at month 7 [13, 15]. The per-protocol analysis group was defined by those who received three full doses of vaccine during the pre-specified visit intervals and provided the 7-month serum sample for assessment of the immunogenicity. The antibody response was measured by geometric mean titre (GMT), and the non-inferiority margin by a 2.0-fold decrease in phase IIB [13]. While the standard is often used as an arithmetic mean that involves taking the sum of group of numbers and then dividing the sum by the count of the numbers, geometric mean is used in data analysis for immunogenicity (e.g., the ability of the vaccine to provoke an immune response and produce HPV neutralising antibodies) [16]. Geometric mean is preferable, as the antibody titres (may be viewed as antibody concentrations) are often non-linear [16]. Geometric mean is calculated by multiplying each observation, then taking the nth root of the product. Assuming a true GMT ratio of 0.80 (9-valent:4-valent) with a standard deviation (SD) of 1.2, the study would have an overall statistical power with one-sided type I error rate of 0.0247 for each pairwise comparison.

For phase III, a per-protocol comparison of the rate of high-grade cervical, vulvar, or vaginal disease related to HPV strains not covered by 4-valent HPV vaccines (HPV-31, -33, -45, -52, and -58) was used as the primary analysis [13]. The target sample size was determined at 14,000 patients (7,000 per group) for the final analysis being targeted when there were at least 30 events observed in the trial [13]. Vaccine efficacy was defined by relative risk reduction (calculated by 1 − risk ratio in 9-valent vaccine/risk ratio in 4-valent vaccine). The target efficacy was defined by having a minimum threshold of 25% in the lower boundary of the 95% confidence interval of the vaccine efficacy. Assuming a true vaccine efficacy of 83% in favour of 9-valent HPV vaccine, a target of 30 events would provide 90% power to demonstrate the target efficacy of 25%. As a key secondary analysis, a non-inferiority testing of the same immunogenicity endpoint was used but with a narrower non-inferiority margin of a 1.5-fold decrease in phase III versus a 2.0-fold decrease that was used in phase IIB. With such a margin, a statistically significant non-inferiority finding would require the lower boundary of the 95% confidence interval for the difference in percentage points to be greater than −5% [13].

Findings

In phase IIB, the analysis of 1,240 patients based on immunological endpoints resulted in selecting the medium-dose 9-valent vaccine, which was thereafter seamlessly tested in phase III in this adaptive trial [13]. For each arm, there were 310 evaluable patients including the selected medium-dose 9-valent vaccine. The data from the phase IIB were combined with the subsequent patients who were later enrolled in phase III after the trial seamlessly transitioned into its confirmatory phase [14]. Between 26 September 2007 and 18 December 2009, a total of 14,215 patients were randomly assigned at a 1:1 ratio to 9-valent vaccine ($n = 7,106$) or to the control 4-valent vaccine ($n = 7,109$) [14]. The per-protocol analysis was performed based on 6,862 patients (96.6%) who completed the protocol for 9-valent vaccine and 6,842 (96.4%) in the 4-valent vaccine control. In comparison to the control vaccine, 9-valent vaccine showed an efficacy of 97.4% (95% CI: 85.0, 99.9%) for high-grade cervical, vulvar, and vaginal disease related to HPV-31, -33, -45, -52, and -58 [14]. The 9-valent vaccine showed incidence rate of 0.5 cases per 10,000 person-years and 19.0 cases per 10,000 person-years in the 4-valent control vaccine group. The 9-valent vaccine also showed non-inferior immunogenic response to HPV-6, -11, -16, and -18 in comparison to the control [13].

For testing of 9-valent vaccine, continuing seamlessly from the exploratory (IIB) to confirmatory (III) phase saved time and resources while enabling the trial's overall goal of confirming the efficacy, immunogenicity, and safety of the 9-valent vaccine. While the overall sample size saved was relatively small at ~620 patients with the seamless design, the investigators have estimated that the follow-up data from phase IIB contributed to at least 10% of the total person-years follow-up [15]. In addition to time efficiency, savings in resources and efforts from not having to establish the trial infrastructure and close them out on two separate occasions should be appreciated. In the early phase portion of the trial, patient recruitment and follow-up procedures could be tested for logistical efficiency for the overall trial [15].

Sample Size Re-Assessment Design

Case Study 9.4: VALOR (NCT01191801)

Background

Vosaroxin and Ara-c combination evaLuating Overall survival in Relapsed/refractory acute myeloid leukaemia (VALOR) was a phase III, double-blinded, adaptive randomised trial that evaluated vosaroxin + cytarabine versus placebo + cytarabine in patients with first relapsed or refractory acute myeloid leukaemia (AML) (NCT01191801) [17]. The relapsed or refractory AML has poor prognosis with median survival that is generally less than 1 year [18]. Before VALOR began, a phase II trial on vosaroxin + cytarabine showed promising early results that supported the initiation of phase III evaluation [19]. While it is often the case that phase II data are used to plan phase III confirmatory trials, it is important to note that estimates from phase II can be subject to uncertainty. This makes planning difficult for phase III trials, especially when there are financial constraints. In this case study, we discuss how a method for adaptive sample size re-assessment called a 'promising zone design' developed by Mehta and Pocock [20] was used to plan and execute VALOR.

Design and Methods

VALOR is an event-driven randomised trial that randomised AML patients 1:1 to the vosaroxin arm or to the placebo [17]. The primary endpoint was overall survival (OS) with the intention-to-treat principle being used as the primary analysis. The initial accrual target was set at 375 deaths in 450 patients based on available phase II data that suggested that an improvement in median OS from 5 months in the placebo group to 7 months in the treatment group could be expected [17, 19]. The initial target would provide 90% power at 5.0% two-sided type I error rate to detect such improvement, which translated to a hazard ratio (HR) of 0.71 (5/7 = 0.71).

As part of a promising zone design, one interim analysis was planned after 173 events, approximately half of the targeted events (Table 9.3). At the interim analysis, the trial could stop early for superiority or futility (option 1a/1b), continue as planned (option 2), or increase the target events (375 to 562 events) and sample size (450 to 675 patients) by 50% (option 3). If the calculated test statistic showed a p-value that was 0.0015 (one-sided), a threshold defined by the O'Brien–Fleming stopping boundary, the trial could stop early for superiority. Conditional power was calculated to potentially allow

Table 9.3 Decision rules for interim analysis in VALOR [17]

Zone	Threshold	Possible decision options at interim analysis[*]
Efficacy zone	One-sided p-value of 0.0015 or lower (defined by O'Brien–Fleming boundary)	Option 1A) Stop trial early for superiority
Favourable zone	Conditional power greater than 90%	Option 2) Continue trial as planned
Promising zone	Conditional power between 30% and 90%	Option 3) Increase sample size and events by 50%
Unfavourable zone	Conditional power between 10% and 30%	Option 2) Continue trial as planned
Futility zone	Conditional power less than 10%	Option 1B) Stop trial early for futility

[*] An interim analysis conducted after 173 events, approximately 50% of the initial target events

for sample size reassessment if the therapy fell in the pre-specified promising zone [20]. In VALOR, conditional power with a maximum number of 562 events and sample size of 675 was calculated assuming the treatment effect observed at the interim was a true effect [17]. If the conditional power was greater than 90%, the treatment was considered to be in the favourable zone where the trial could continue onto the initial target events and sample size [17]. If the conditional fell between 30% and 90%, this was considered the promising zone where the target number of events and sample size would be increased by 50%. If the conditional power was between 10% and 30% (unfavourable zone), it did not warrant a sample size increase since the sample size would need to be increased beyond what is feasible to recruit to ensure adequate conditional power. If the conditional power was less than 10%, the trial could stop early for futility because the treatment would be a lost cause.

Findings

The interim analysis was conducted at 173 events. The independent DSMB recommended continuation of the VALOR trial with an increase in sample size [17]. Vosaroxin fell in the promising zone with conditional power of 82% [17]. The final analysis was conducted with a total of 711 patients who were enrolled between 16 December 2010 and 25 September 2013 (356 to vosaroxin and 355 to placebo) [17]. The median OS was 7.5 months (95% CI: 6.4, 8.5) for vosaroxin and 6.1 months (95% CI: 5.2, 7.1) for placebo. The trial barely missed its primary goal of demonstrating a statistically significant improvement in OS with an HR of 0.87 (95% CI: 0.73, 1.02) with a two-sided p-value of 0.0610 [17]. However, a predefined secondary analysis that accounted for factors used to define stratum for randomisation (stratified log-rank test) showed a significant HR of 0.81 (95% CI: 0.67, 0.97) with a p-value of 0.0241, suggesting a statistically significant improvement in OS [17].

It is important consider feasibility constraints that exist for clinical trial research. VALOR was sponsored by a small biotech company, so it was not feasible for them to make upfront financial commitments in the planning stage. Sample size re-assessment procedures, such as the promising zone that we discussed for this case study, can help balance cost and time to de-risk investment in clinical trial research [21]. VALOR is a high-quality adaptive clinical trial from the standpoint of the study design and implementation. Albeit barely, VALOR did miss its goal of achieving statistical significance for its primary endpoint. In the end, adaptive trial designs are used to manage uncertainty, but they cannot eliminate uncertainty altogether. It is not possible to design a study that can guarantee success, but for right questions, we can plan for data-driven ways to minimise our anticipated regret (see Chapter 1).

Response Adaptive Randomisation Design

Case Study 9.5: RACE (NCT01665092)

Background

Rapid Administration of Carnitine in sEpsis (RACE) was a phase IIB, placebo-controlled randomised clinical trial with Bayesian response adaptive randomisation designed to assess the efficacy of L-carnitine in reduction in the Sequential Organ Failure Assessment (SOFA) score for patients with septic shock (NCT01665092) [22]. As L-carnitine has been shown to improve the adverse haemodynamic effects of sepsis, the RACE trial investigators hypothesised that early adjunctive L-carnitine administration in vasopressor-dependent septic shock patients could reduce cumulative organ failure at 48 hours, measured by the SOFA score and 28-day mortality [23]. Three doses of L-carnitine were compared against placebo in this phase IIB trial in order to find the most effective dose that could be tested in a phase III trial [22].

Design and Methods

Patients could randomly be assigned to one of three active treatment arms or the placebo arm [22]. The active treatment arms consisted of low (6 g), medium (12 g), or high (18 g) doses of L-carnitine administered intravenously for 12 hours [22]. The primary endpoint was a change in the SOFA scores from baseline to 48 hours where negative change in scores indicated a clinical improvement. A key secondary endpoint of this trial included 28-day mortality. The target sample size for this trial was 250 patients, where approximately one-third of the allocation would be maintained to the placebo arm. Response adaptive randomisation could be used to adapt the allocation in the remaining two-thirds of the allocation between the three doses of L-carnitine (Table 9.4).

For the L-carnitine study arms, the allocation ratio was preferentially adapted based on the probability of each dose being the best dose for improving SOFA scores. There was an initial burn-in period of 40 patients that used a fixed allocation of 1:1:1:1. Interim analyses were conducted on every 12 patients to adapt the allocation ratios between the treatment arms until the target enrolment or until a stopping rule was met, whichever came first. There were stopping rules for futility and superiority. The trial could stop early for futility if the most promising L-carnitine dose showed less than 40% posterior probability that it led to an improvement in SOFA score in comparison to the placebo. For superiority threshold, predictive probability of an eventual success was calculated with success being defined as achieving statistical significance for 28-day mortality endpoint in a subsequent phase III two-arm randomised trial with an enrolment target of 2,000 patients (1:1 to control or selected dose of L-carnitine). The trial could be stopped early for superiority, if the most promising dose had a greater than 90% posterior probability that it led to an improvement in SOFA score in comparison to the placebo and a predictive probability of success that was greater than 70%.

Table 9.4 Decision rules for interim analysis in RACE [22]

Adaptations

Burn-in period:

Fixed allocation (1:1:1:1) for 40 patients

Post burn-in period:

Interim analyses every 12 patients up to 250 patients or a stopping rule

Response adaptive randomisation	~One-third fixed allocation maintained to control ~Two-thirds of allocation can be adapted to the best dose[*]
Early stopping for futility	<40% posterior probability that the most promising dose leads to improvement in SOFA at 48 hours versus placebo
Early stopping for superiority	>90% posterior probability that the most promising dose leads to improvement in SOFA at 48 hours versus placebo & >70% predictive probability of success[**]

[*] Allocation adapted based on probability of each dose being the best dose for improving SOFA scores.
[**] For the calculation of predictive probability of success, success was defined by achieving statistical significance (p-value < 0.025) for the 28-day mortality endpoint in a subsequent phase III randomised trial with 1:1 allocation and 2,000 patient enrolment target.

The trial was considered to have positive findings, if at least one of the doses had 90% posterior probability of greater improvement in SOFA scores at 48 hours versus placebo, and also if there was at least 30% predictive probability of phase III success based on the 28-day mortality endpoint. Trial simulations were used to calibrate the decision rules to have optimal operating characteristics. Based on simulation that was repeated 30,000 times, enrolling up to 250 patients under the pre-specified rules for response adaptive randomisation and early stopping had an overall type I error rate of 4.3% [22]. If the low, medium, and high doses of L-carnitine had treatment effects of 0, −1, and −2 with respect to the change in SOFA scores versus the placebo arm, the simulations showed a statistical power of 91.1%.

Findings

Between 5 March 2013 and 5 February 2018, 250 septic shock patients were enrolled into the RACE trial [22]. During the burn-in period of 40 patients, 10 patients were randomly assigned to each study arm (Table 9.5). After the burn-in period, 31% ($n = 65/210$) of patients were assigned to the control group as approximately one-third of the allocation was maintained to the control; 45.7% ($n = 96/210$) were preferentially allocated to the high-dose arm over the medium-dose (11.4%; $n = 24/210$) and the low-dose (11.9%; $n = 25/210$). Overall, out of 250 patients who were randomised in this trial, 30.0% ($n = 75/250$) were randomly assigned to the placebo, 14.0% ($n = 35/250$) to low-dose, 13.6% ($n = 34/250$) to medium-dose, and 42.4% ($n = 106/250$) to the high-dose.

In the intention-to-treat analysis, the mean (SD) changes in the SOFA score for the low-, medium-, and high-dose groups were −1.27 (SD: 0.49), −1.66 (SD: 0.38), and −1.97 (SD: 0.32), respectively, versus −1.63 (SD: 0.35) in the placebo group (Table 9.5). The high-dose arm, which had the best SOFA scores, had a 78% posterior probability of being superior to the placebo arm. The high-dose arm also had the highest predictive probability of phase III success at 40%. While this was higher than 30% predictive probability of success that was pre-specified (40% > 30%), the trial did not end up meeting its pre-specified criteria for success, as the high-dose arm had a posterior probability of success that was lower than the 90% a priori threshold (78% < 90%).

Table 9.5 Summary of the RACE trial[*] [22]

Summary	Low-dose arm	Medium-dose arm	High-dose arm	Placebo	Total
Randomisation during the burn-in period: N (%)	10 (25.0%)	10 (25.0%)	10 (25.0%)	10 (25.0%)	40 (100%)
Randomisation after the burn-in period: N (%)	25 (11.9%)	24 (11.4%)	96 (45.7%)	65 (31.0%)	210 (100%)
Overall randomisation: N (%)	35 (14.0%)	34 (13.6%)	106 (42.4%)	75 (30.0%)	250 (100%)
Change in SOFA scores: Mean (SD)	−1.27 (SD: 0.49)	−1.66 (SD: 0.38)	−1.97 (SD: 0.32)	−1.63 (SD: 0.35)	−
Posterior probability of being superior to placebo	24%	54%	78%	−	−
Mortality at 28 days: N (%)	20/34 (58.8%)	16/32 (50%)	45/104 (43.3%)	34/74 (45.9%)	115/247 (46.6%)
Predictive probability of phase III success	10%	22%	40%	−	−

[*] Intention-to-treat analysis results on efficacy endpoints and probability of superiority/success are presented in this table.
SD = standard deviation

Adaptive Enrichment Design

Case Study 9.6: TAPPAS (NCT02979899)

Background

A randomised phase III trial of Trc105 And Pazopanib versus Pazopanib alone in patients with advanced AngioSarcoma (TAPPAS) was an adaptive enrichment, randomised trial that assessed the efficacy of carotuximab + pazopanib (treatment) versus pazopanib alone (control) in patients with angiosarcoma [26, 27]. Prior to TAPPAS, carotuximab combined with pazopanib had shown promising results for cutaneous angiosarcoma in an exploratory, single-arm trial [26]. The trial started with recruiting a broad population of angiosarcoma patients with both cutaneous and non-cutaneous sub-types. As there was an indication for possible benefit of carotuximab + pazopanib being targeted for cutaneous angiosarcoma, TAPPAS used an adaptive trial design that could allow for sample size re-assessment or population enrichment to cutaneous angiosarcoma at the planned interim analysis [26, 27].

Design and Methods

TAPPAS used a stratified permuted block randomisation at an equal allocation ratio (1:1) to the treatment or to the control arm [26]. Patients were stratified by angiosarcoma type (cutaneous vs. non-cutaneous) and by the number of prior systemic therapy (0 vs. 1–2) with varying block sizes of 2 or 4. The primary analysis was based on the statistical comparison of progression-free survival (PFS) based on the intention-to-treat principle. The initial target was set at 95 events with enrolment of 190 patients for 83% power at 5% two-sided alpha to detect an overall HR of 0.55 for an improvement of median PFS from 4 months (control) to 7.27 months (treatment).

An enrichment design was used due to possible heterogeneity of treatment effect between cutaneous and non-cutaneous angiosarcoma sub-type. For this, an interim analysis was planned after observing 40 events or 30 days after the 120th patient has been enrolled, whichever came first. Assuming the treatment effect observed at the interim analysis as true effect, conditional power of demonstrating significant treatment effect for the full population (CP-full) and for the cutaneous angiosarcoma (CP-cutaneous) were calculated to define the favourable, promising, enrichment, and unfavourable zones (Table 9.6). The trial was considered to fall into the favourable zone if the CP-full was greater than 95%. The trial in the favourable zone would continue as planned and enrol 190 more patients, and the final analysis would be conducted after 95 events have been observed. Having the CP-full between 30% and 95% was considered as the promising zone; in this case, the enrolment target for the overall population would be increased to 340 patients, and the final analysis would be conducted after 170 events have been observed. The trial fell in the enrichment zone if the CP-full was less than 30% and the CP-cutaneous was greater than 50%. In the case of the enrichment zone, the trial would restrict the enrolment to cutaneous angiosarcoma only, where 160 cutaneous patients would be enrolled with the final analysis being performed after 110 events observed from the cutaneous group. If in the unfavourable zone, defined by CP-full being less than 30% and the CP-cutaneous being 50% or less, the trial would continue

Table 9.6 Decision rules for interim analysis in TAPPAS [26, 27]

Zone	Threshold	Possible decision options[*]
Favourable zone	CP-full >95%	Option 1) Continue as planned to 190 patients and 95 events
Promising zone	CP-full 30% to 95%	Option 2) Increase enrolment target from 190 patients and 95 events to 340 patients and 170 events
Enrichment zone	CP-full <30% and CP-cutaneous >50%	Option 3) Enrich and enrol 160 cutaneous patients only thereafter for a final analysis done at 110 events in the enriched group
Unfavourable zone	CP-full <0% and CP-cutaneous ≤50%	Option 1) Continue as planned to 190 patients and 95 events
Futility zone	Up to the judgment of the independent DSMB	Option 4) End the trial for futility

[*] An interim analysis conducted after 40 events or 30 days after the 120th patient has been enrolled

as originally planned as with the favourable zone. The DSMB could have recommended termination for futility based on their judgment, if the treatment arm was doing worse than the control group. For futility stopping, there was no formal pre-specified rule defined in TAPPS.

Findings

The latest publication out of the TAPPAS trial included the interim analysis results by Jones et al., 2022 [26]. For the interim analysis, a total of 123 patients were enrolled, with 62 patients randomised to treatment and 61 patients to the control arm between 16 February 2017 and 12 April 2019 [26]. The primary analysis for the interim analysis included the full population of both cutaneous and non-cutaneous angiosarcoma patients. There were no important differences of PFS between the treatment and the control group (HR: 0.98; 95% CI: 0.51, 1.84; p-value = 0.95). The treatment arm had a median PFS of 4.2 months (95% CI, 2.8, 8.3 months), and the control arm had a median PFS of 4.3 months (95% CI: 2.9 months, upper interval not reached).

There were 64 patients with cutaneous angiosarcoma available for the interim analysis; however, the treatment arm did not show important differences for PFS compared to the control arm for the hypothesised group [26]. Among the cutaneous angiosarcoma sub-type, the treatment arm had a median PFS of 4.2 months (95% CI: 2.8, 8.3 months) and the control arm had a median PFS of 5.6 months (95% CI: 2.6, 5.6 months). The HR for PFS was 1.07 (95% CI: 0.43, 2.67; p-value = .89).

In this trial, the treatment arm did not show improvement in PFS versus the control arm in either the full population or the cutaneous sub-type [26]. This case study is an important example of the extension of the promising zone method that is usually used for sample size re-assessment for adaptive enrichment design [20, 27]. Despite being designed as an enrichment design, the TAPPAS trial did not meet the threshold for enrichment zone. As the trial did not show any benefits for carotuximab + pazopanib, the trial ended early based on futility.

References

1. Zajicek JP, Hobart JC, Slade A, et al. Multiple sclerosis and extract of cannabis: results of the MUSEC trial. *J Neurol Neurosurg Psychiatry*. 2012;**83**(11):1125–32.

2. Bethoux F, Marrie RA. A cross-sectional study of the impact of spasticity on daily activities in multiple sclerosis. *Patient*. 2016;**9**(6):537–46.

3. O'Brien PC, Fleming TR. A multiple testing procedure for clinical trials. *Biometrics*. 1979;**35**(3):549–56.

4. Dimairo M, Pallmann P, Wason J, et al. The Adaptive designs CONSORT Extension (ACE) statement: a checklist with explanation and elaboration guideline for reporting randomised trials that use an adaptive design. *BMJ*. 2020;**369**:m115.

5. Dimairo M, Pallmann P, Wason J, et al. The adaptive designs CONSORT extension (ACE) statement: a checklist with explanation and elaboration guideline for reporting randomised trials that use an adaptive design. *Trials*. 2020;**21**(1):528.

6. Sevransky JE, Rothman RE, Hager DN, et al. Effect of vitamin C, thiamine, and hydrocortisone on ventilator- and vasopressor-free days in patients with sepsis: the VICTAS randomized clinical trial. *JAMA*. 2021;**325**(8):742–50.

7. Lindsell CJ, McGlothlin A, Nwosu S, et al. Update to the Vitamin C, Thiamine and Steroids in Sepsis (VICTAS) protocol: statistical analysis plan for a prospective, multicenter, double-blind, adaptive

sample size, randomized, placebo-controlled, clinical trial. *Trials.* 2019;**20**(1):670.

8. Hager DN, Hooper MH, Bernard GR, et al. The Vitamin C, Thiamine and Steroids in Sepsis (VICTAS) Protocol: a prospective, multi-center, double-blind, adaptive sample size, randomized, placebo-controlled, clinical trial. *Trials.* 2019;**20**(1):197.

9. Bauchner H, Fontanarosa PB, Golub RM. Funding and DSMB membership in the VICTAS clinical trial. *JAMA.* 2021;**325**(8):751–2.

10. Galloway DA, Laimins LA. Human papillomaviruses: shared and distinct pathways for pathogenesis. *Curr Opin Virol.* 2015;**14**:87–92.

11. Plummer M, de Martel C, Vignat J, et al. Global burden of cancers attributable to infections in 2012: a synthetic analysis. *Lancet Glob Health.* 2016;**4**(9):e609–16.

12. Joura EA, Leodolter S, Hernandez-Avila M, et al. Efficacy of a quadrivalent prophylactic human papillomavirus (types 6, 11, 16, and 18) L1 virus-like-particle vaccine against high-grade vulval and vaginal lesions: a combined analysis of three randomised clinical trials. *Lancet.* 2007;**369**(9574):1693–702.

13. Joura EA, Giuliano AR, Iversen OE, et al. A 9-valent HPV vaccine against infection and intraepithelial neoplasia in women. *N Engl J Med.* 2015;**372**(8):711–23.

14. Huh WK, Joura EA, Giuliano AR, et al. Final efficacy, immunogenicity, and safety analyses of a nine-valent human papillomavirus vaccine in women aged 16–26 years: a randomised, double-blind trial. *Lancet.* 2017;**390**(10108):2143–59.

15. Chen YH, Gesser R, Luxembourg A. A seamless phase IIB/III adaptive outcome trial: design rationale and implementation challenges. *Clin Trials.* 2015;**12**(1):84–90.

16. Reverberi R. The statistical analysis of immunohaematological data. *Blood Transfus.* 2008;**6**(1):37–45.

17. Ravandi F, Ritchie EK, Sayar H, et al. Vosaroxin plus cytarabine versus placebo plus cytarabine in patients with first relapsed or refractory acute myeloid leukaemia (VALOR): a randomised, controlled, double-blind, multinational, phase 3 study. *Lancet Oncol.* 2015;**16**(9):1025–36.

18. Breems DA, Van Putten WL, Huijgens PC, et al. Prognostic index for adult patients with acute myeloid leukemia in first relapse. *J Clin Oncol.* 2005;**23**(9):1969–78.

19. Lancet JE, Roboz GJ, Cripe LD, et al. A phase 1b/2 study of vosaroxin in combination with cytarabine in patients with relapsed or refractory acute myeloid leukemia. *Haematologica.* 2015;**100**(2):231–7.

20. Mehta CR, Pocock SJ. Adaptive increase in sample size when interim results are promising: a practical guide with examples. *Stat Med.* 2011;**30**(28):3267–84.

21. David FS, Bobulsky S, Schulz K, Patel N. Creating value with financially adaptive clinical trials. *Nat Rev Drug Discov.* 2015;**14**(8):523–4.

22. Jones AE, Puskarich MA, Shapiro NI, et al. Effect of levocarnitine vs placebo as an adjunctive treatment for septic shock: the Rapid Administration of Carnitine in Sepsis (RACE) randomized clinical trial. *JAMA Netw Open.* 2018;**1**(8):e186076.

23. Calvani M, Reda E, Arrigoni-Martelli E. Regulation by carnitine of myocardial fatty acid and carbohydrate metabolism under normal and pathological conditions. *Basic Res Cardiol.* 2000;**95**(2):75–83.

24. Krams M, Lees KR, Hacke W, et al. Acute Stroke Therapy by Inhibition of Neutrophils (ASTIN): an adaptive dose-response study of UK-279,276 in acute ischemic stroke. *Stroke.* 2003;**34**(11):2543–8.

25. Grieve AP, Krams M. ASTIN: a Bayesian adaptive dose-response trial in acute stroke. *Clin Trials.* 2005;**2**(4):340–51.

26. Jones RL, Ravi V, Brohl AS, et al. Efficacy and safety of TRC105 plus pazopanib vs pazopanib alone for treatment of patients with advanced angiosarcoma: a randomized clinical trial. *JAMA Oncol.* 2022;**8**(5):740–7.

27. Mehta CR, Liu L, Theuer C. An adaptive population enrichment phase III trial of TRC105 and pazopanib versus pazopanib alone in patients with advanced angiosarcoma (TAPPAS trial). *Ann Oncol.* 2019;**30**(1):103–8.

Chapter 1

Case Studies of Platform Trials

Jay J. H. Park, J. Kyle Wathen, and Edward J. Mills

Introduction

In this chapter, we discuss four adaptive randomised platform trials as case studies: Systemic Therapy in Advancing or Metastatic Prostate Cancer: Evaluation of Drug Efficacy (STAMPEDE); Investigation of Serial studies to Predict Your Therapeutic Response with Imaging and Molecular Analysis 2 (I-SPY 2); Randomised Evaluation of COVID-19 Therapy (RECOVERY); and TOGETHER. The two longest ongoing platform trials, STAMPEDE and I-SPY 2, are widely considered to be the two hallmark trials [1]. RECOVERY and TOGETHER are another two important examples of ongoing platform trials conducted for COVID-19 [2].

Case Study 10.1: STAMPEDE (NCT00268476)

Background

Systemic Therapy in Advancing or Metastatic Prostate Cancer: Evaluation of Drug Efficacy (STAMPEDE; NCT00268476) is a multi-arm, multi-stage (MAMS) platform randomised trial evaluating multiple treatment options for men with advanced or metastatic prostate cancer starting long-term androgen deprivation therapy (ADT), a type of hormone therapy [3–5]. STAMPEDE is the first platform trial to be conducted after being launched for recruitment in the UK on 8 July 2005 [1, 3–5]. This platform trial has remained active for close to 20 years and has included 10 interventions for advanced prostate cancer patients with complete evaluations of eight therapies and two currently active in the trial (Table 10.1) [3–5]. According to their U.S. National Library of Medicine ClinicalTrials.gov record, it is intended to continue at least until December 2030 [6].

When STAMPEDE began, it was first described as a multi-arm, multi-stage (MAMS) design [4, 5]. STAMPEDE started using the term 'multi-arm, multi-stage, platform design' in 2016 [12] after two U.S.-based scientists, Mary Redman and Carmen Allegra [13], first published the concept of master protocol in 2015. MAMS, first described in 2003, refers to a type of sequential design that applies to multi-arm clinical trials [14]. In MAMS design, multiple intervention arms can be evaluated against a common control arm using multiple analyses [3, 4, 14, 15]. The features of MAMS design have many similarities to adaptive platform randomised trials; in fact, platform trials have been considered as an extension of MAMS design, as multiple interventions ('multi-arm') undergoing multiple interim evaluations ('multi-stage') are part of the their design features [15, 16]. However, it should be noted that adaptive platform randomised trials have additional flexibilities of allowing new interventions that were not pre-specified in the design to be added and even the standard-of-care to be updated over time [16, 17].

Table 10.1 A list of interventions that entered STAMPEDE, as of April 2022 [6]

Interventions	Start time	End time
1. Zoledronic acid [7]	5 Oct 2005	13 March 2013
2. Docetaxel + prednisolone [7]	5 Oct 2005	13 March 2013
3. Celecoxib [8]	5 Oct 2005	6 April 2011
4. Zoledronic acid + docetaxel + prednisolone [7]	5 Oct 2005	13 March 2013
5. Zoledronic acid + celecoxib [8]	5 Oct 2005	6 April 2011
6. Abiraterone + prednisolone [9]	15 Nov 2011	17 Jan 2014
7. M1 radiotherapy [10]	22 Jan 2013	2 Sept 2016
8. Abiraterone + enzalutamide + prednisolone [11]	29 July 2014	31 March 2016
9. Metformin	June 2016	Active for recruitment
10. Transdermal oestradiol	Dec 2018	Active for recruitment

Design and Methods

STAMPEDE is an adaptive, seamless phase IIB/III, MAMS, platform randomised trial [4, 5, 18, 19]. For each intervention, there are three interim analyses that allowed for early stopping based on futility and a final statistical analysis that aimed to confirm the efficacy of each intervention. The interim analyses are based on failure-free survival (FFS), whereas the final analysis is based on overall survival (OS). The investigators justified the use of FFS as a surrogate outcome for OS under the assumptions that an improvement or little-to-no change in FFS would correspondingly lead to an improvement or little-to-no change on OS [5]. A larger number of FFS events than deaths could be expected; however, since the magnitude of treatment effects on FFS is largely greater than OS, a larger magnitude of hazard ratio (HR) was targeted for FFS than the primary outcome of OS [5].

STAMPEDE is an event-based trial in which the interim and final analyses are triggered based on the predefined number of events. At each interim analysis, the decision to drop the intervention or progress them onto the next stage (interim analysis) is made using frequentist stopping rules [19]. For each intervention arm, the first futility interim analysis is conducted when there are 114 FFS events observed in the concurrent control arm, 214 FFS events for second futility analysis, and 334 FFS events for the third futility analysis [19]. To avoid inadvertently dropping an experimental arm that may prove to be effective, early stages were designed with higher power (lower type II error) and alpha. For the first interim analysis, experimental arms must have demonstrated an HR point estimate of less than 1.00 for FFS compared against the concurrent control to progress onto the next stage. The HRs of 0.92 and 0.89 are used for the second and third interim analyses, respectively. The final analysis, if required, uses a one-sided significance level of 0.025 based on OS. The overall one-sided type I error across the four analyses for the pairwise comparisons was calculated at approximately 0.013 [5, 18, 19].

Findings

When STAMPEDE first began in 2005, it started as a six-arm trial with five intervention arms being compared against a common control arm [3, 4]. Unequal allocation ratios in favour of the control group of 2:1:1:1:1:1 was used initially to maximise overall statistical power across multiple pairwise comparisons against the common control arm. Since the start, five new intervention arms have been added into the platform with the first intervention (intervention 6) being added on 15 November 2011 (Table 10.1). STAMPEDE had started to operate with less active arms, so the allocation was reduced to an equal ratio between different intervention and control arms [9–11]. Several scientific and practical considerations have been made to guide decisions to introduce new intervention arms [19]. These include a sound rationale, supported by both a robust biological hypothesis and positive evidence of potential efficacy. Industry partners will be consulted and must have been issued or be near the issuing of necessary licensing.

Over the years, STAMPEDE has generated randomised clinical trial evidence for multiple therapies for prostate cancer research. Notable are their findings on docetaxel. Between 05 October 2005 and 31 March 2013, 592 patients were randomly assigned to the docetaxel arm with an overlapping 1,184 control patients [12]. Addition of docetaxel to standard-of-care was shown to improve survival of these patients with prostate cancer in the STAMPEDE trial. In comparison to the control group, the docetaxel arm showed an HR of 0.61 (95% CI: 0.53, 0.70) for FFS and 0.78 (95% CI: 0.66, 0.93) for overall survival [12]. This was confirmed with a meta-analysis that included other randomised clinical trials, CHAARTED [20] and GETUG-15 [21], which confirmed the individual study finding from STAMPEDE [22]. Based on these findings, the standard-of-care was updated to include docetaxel in STAMPEDE. In clinical trials, there can be instances of internal and/or external scientific discoveries that warrant a change in standard-of-care for the trial. Platform trials, as seen in STAMPEDE, are generally better equipped to accommodate the change in standard-of-care than other conventional (non-platform) trials that are generally considered for a shorter time period [16, 17, 23].

Case Study 10.2: I-SPY 2 (NCT01042379)

Background

Investigation of Serial studies to Predict Your Therapeutic Response with Imaging and Molecular Analysis 2 (I-SPY 2; NCT01042379) is one of the most coveted adaptive platform trials that started before the COVID-19 pandemic [1, 17, 24]. I-SPY 2 is a Bayesian, adaptive platform randomised trial with a response adaptive randomisation design investigating neoadjuvant therapies for women with locally advanced breast cancer [25–27]. I-SPY 2 is a phase IIB trial conducted with an overall goal of identifying candidate-targeted therapies for a given molecular trait (biomarker signature) for future phase III evaluation [27].

Design and Methods

I-SPY 2 is a biomarker-guided trial that used biomarker information for eligibility criteria, stratified randomisation, and assessment of efficacy [27]. Biomarker information on oestrogen receptor (ER), progesterone receptor (PR), human epidermal growth factor receptor 2 (HER2), and MammaPrint scoring (a score based on the activity of 70 genes related to breast cancer) are used as eligibility standards to recruit high-risk breast cancer patients into the study [27–29]. Information on HR (positive vs. negative), HER2 (positive vs negative), and MammaPrint scores (high vs. low) were used to create 8 (= $2 \times 2 \times 2$) strata for stratified randomisation, and the same information was used to create 10 biomarker signatures in which each experimental intervention would be assessed for efficacy [27].

In I-SPY 2, patients with HER2 negative tumours would receive 12 weekly cycles of paclitaxel followed by 4 cycles of doxorubicin and cyclophosphamide every 2 to 3 weeks as standard-of-care. Patients with HER2 positive tumours, on the other hand, would receive 12 weekly cycles of paclitaxel and trastuzumab, followed by 4 cycles of doxorubicin and cyclophosphamide. All patients are required to undergo multiple magnetic resonance imaging (MRI) examinations (baseline, 3 weeks, and 12 weeks after starting paclitaxel therapy), core biopsy examination at baseline, and surgery at the end of treatment cycle in which the primary outcome of pathological complete response (CR) would be assessed. In I-SPY 2, interventions combined with standard chemotherapy are evaluated against the standard chemotherapy alone (control arm) for each of these 10 signatures.

Regimens in this trial are evaluated within 10 biomarker signature sub-groups for the goal matching therapies based on the genetic characteristics of the breast cancer. The primary objective of this trial is to determine the predictive probability of success in a subsequent phase III trial for each regimen based on the CR outcome for each biomarker signature sub-group. The decision to graduate or drop a targeted therapy is based on its performance in these 10 pre-specified biomarker signatures. Within each molecular sub-type, 20% of patients would be assigned to the control and the remaining 80% were distributed using response adaptive randomisation that was based on the probability of each therapy being the most effective therapy for that given sub-type [27]. For each intervention, the maximum target sample size was generally set at 120 patients with a burn-in period of 20 patients, meaning interventions with fewer than 20 patients would have a fixed allocation instead of the allocation determined using response adaptive randomisation [27].

The stopping for superiority is defined by a graduation of the therapy onto a phase III trial evaluation for the given biomarker signature; whereas stopping for futility is determined based on lack-of-efficacy for all 10 biomarker signatures [27]. The decision rules for superiority and futility were based on Bayesian predictive probability of being successful in a future phase III trial that is calculated assuming a randomised clinical trial with an equal allocation of 300 patients. The decision rule for superiority (graduation), defined as a sufficiently high level (85%) of predictive probability for a given biomarker signature, could be made when at least 60 patients are assigned to that therapy. The decision rule for futility, defined by predictive probability that is less than 10% in all 10 signatures for a given therapy, could be made when there are at least 20 patients assigned to the therapy. The simulations for I-SPY 2 showed that such typical design had at least 80% power for a given biomarker signature and at least log odds of 1.5 for CR in comparison to the control, and the overall type I error rate was generally less than 10%.

Findings

Since being launched on 1 March 2010, I-SPY 2 has included close to 30 interventions (Table 10.2). According to U.S. National Library of Medicine ClinicalTrials.Gov, it is intended to continue at least until December 2031 [30]. There have been several targeted therapies that have graduated from I-SPY 2 [31]. For instance, a poly-ADP ribose polymerase inhibitor, veliparib-carboplatin, graduated on December 2013 for triple negative breast cancer (HER2, HR, and MP negative) after showing an 88% predictive probability of being successful in an eventual phase III trial [26]. Neratinib, a tyrosine kinase inhibitor, also graduated on December 2013 for HER2+/HR− breast cancer [25]. There are examples of other targeted therapies that have graduated for various biomarker signatures, including MK-2206 (AKT inhibitor); trastuzumab emtansine + pertuzumab (HER2 dimerisation inhibitor); pertuzumab + paclitaxel + herceptin (HER2/neu receptor antagonist); and pembrolizumab + paclitaxel + doxorubicin + cyclophosphamide (PD-1 inhibitor) [31-33].

Table 10.2 A list of interventions that entered I-SPY 2, as of April 2022 [30]

Interventions

1. Standard therapy (control)
2. AMG 386 with or without trastuzumab
3. AMG 479 (Ganitumab) plus metformin
4. MK-2206 with or without trastuzumab
5. AMG 386 and trastuzumab
6. T-DM1 and pertuzumab
7. Pertuzumab and trastuzumab
8. Ganetespib
9. Veliparib-carboplatin (ABT-888) [26]
10. Neratinib
11. Plx3397
12. Pembrolizumab – 4 cycle
13. Talazoparib plus irinotecan
14. Patritumab and trastuzumab
15. Pembrolizumab – 8 cycle
16. Sgn-liv1a
17. Durvalumab plus olaparib
18. Sd-101 + pembrolizumab
19. Tucatinib
20. Cemiplimab
21. Cemiplimab plus REGN3767
22. Trilaciclib with or without trastuzumab + pertuzumab
23. SYD985 ([vic-]trastuzumab duocarmazine)
24. Oral Paclitaxel + encequidar + dostarlimab (TSR-042) + carboplatin with or without trastuzumab
25. Oral Paclitaxel + encequidar + dostarlimab (TSR-042) with or without trastuzumab
26. Amcenestrant monotherapy
27. Amcenestrant + abemaciclib
28. Amcenestrant + letrozole

The list of interventions is from U.S. National Library of Medicine ClinicalTrials.gov record of I-SPY 2, NCT01042379 on 27 April 2022.

Case Study 10.3: RECOVERY (ISRCTN50189673 & NCT04381936)

Background

Randomised Evaluation of COVID-19 Therapy (RECOVERY; ISRCTN50189673 & NCT04381936) is one of the most famous clinical trials from the COVID-19 pandemic [23, 34–38]. This UK-based, large platform randomised trial has evaluated multiple different interventions for hospitalised COVID-19 patients against the usual standard-of-care across several hundred hospitals in the UK. RECOVERY is perhaps most well known for being the first randomised clinical trial during the COVID-19 pandemic to discover a life-saving treatment in dexamethasone [39]. The results that were first made public as a press release, a pre-print, and then a publication produced a large increase in the administration of corticosteroid overnight among hospitalised patients who required oxygen [39].

Between the time that the first patient was randomised on 19 March 2020 to when dexamethasone was announced to the world as a life-saving treatment for COVID-19 on 16 June 2020, the trial was able to rapidly recruit over 12,000 patients in a short span of ~4 months [39–41]. Such rapid recruitment for the RECOVERY trial was made possible due to unprecedented leadership and national-level collaborations across the UK as well as the simplicity of the trial. For instance, on 6 May 2020, the UK's four chief medical officers and the NHS England and Improvement's national medical director have written a joint letter to encourage and harmonise efforts to enrol patients into the RECOVERY trial and three other platform trials (i.e., ACCORD, PRINCIPLE, and REMAP-CAP) [42]. To date, RECOVERY has generated convincing evidence on the clinical efficacy of multiple treatments for hospitalised patients with COVID-19 [40, 41, 43–52]. It has gone on to expand recruitment beyond the UK to include several other countries.

Design and Methods

RECOVERY is an adaptive, open-label platform randomised trial with a factorial design [40, 41, 45–52]. As no appropriate information was available to estimate the sample size requirement reliably at the beginning stage and due to rapidly changing conditions throughout the pandemic, sample size and recruitment have been monitored by the steering committee in a blinded fashion. Based on intention-to-treat (as-randomised) principle, the primary analysis involves a pairwise comparison against a concurrent control arm based on 28-day mortality status (yes or no). No formal statistical rules are used. The data monitoring is done by an independent data monitoring committee that is asked to inform the steering committee when they view the study has generated strong enough evidence on each statistical comparisons throughout the trial.

Findings

On 5 June 2020, the RECOVERY trial announced the decision to discontinue the evaluation of hydroxychloroquine (HCQ) due to lack of clinical efficacy [52]. When data from 1,542 patients randomised to HCQ were compared to 3,132 patients randomised to the control group, HCQ did not demonstrate any clinical benefits on 28-day mortality (23.5% in the control group vs. 25.7% in the HCQ group) showing an HR of 1.11 (95% CI: 0.98, 1.26) [52].

On 22 June 2020, the RECOVERY trial published preliminary report findings on low-dose dexamethasone (6 mg once daily for 10 days) as a preprint [44]. The peer-reviewed results became available shortly thereafter [41]. This analysis for dexamethasone included data from 2,104 patients who were randomised to dexamethasone and 4,321 patients who were randomised to the control group. For the overall population, dexamethasone showed age-adjusted relative risk (RR) of 0.83 (95% CI: 0.74, 0.92) for 28-day mortality in comparison to the control group (mortality rate of 21.6% in dexamethasone and 24.6% in the control group). The demonstrated mortality reduction benefits varied among patients who received different respiratory support at randomisation. For instance, dexamethasone did not demonstrate any mortality reduction benefits among patients who did not receive any ventilation support (RR: 1.22; 95% CI: 0.93, 1.61), but for patients who received non-invasive ventilation (RR: 0.80; 95% CI: 0.70, 0.92) and invasive mechanical ventilation (RR: 0.65; 95% CI: 0.51, 0.82), there were important mortality reduction benefits from dexamethasone.

As of today, RECOVERY has included a total of 16 interventions in the trial (Table 10.3). Many of these interventions already have been completed for clinical evaluation. There are several arms currently active (high-dose corticosteroid; empagliflozin; sotrovimab; molnupiravir; and paxlovid). It is likely that there will be more interventions added, but the wide impressive list of different therapies should highlight the important value of establishing a platform trial and a common trial infrastructure for clinical trial research [53].

Table 10.3 A list of interventions that have entered RECOVERY as of April 2022

Interventions

1. Hydroxychloroquine
2. Azithromycin
3. Convalescent plasma
4. Tocilizumab
5. Immunoglobulin
6. Synthetic neutralising antibodies
7. Aspirin
8. Colchicine
9. Baricitinib
10. Anakinra
11. Dimethyl fumarate
12. High-dose corticosteroid (currently active)
13. Empagliflozin (currently active)
14. Sotrovimab (currently active)
15. Molnupiravir (currently active)
16. Paxlovid (currently active)

The list of interventions is from U.S. National Library of Medicine ClinicalTrials.gov record of RECOVERY trial, NCT01042379, on 27 April 2022.

Case Study 10.4: TOGETHER (NCT04727424)

Background

TOGETHER (NCT04727424) is an outpatient adaptive randomised platform trial to evaluate repurposed therapies among symptomatic Brazilian adults with COVID-19 at high risk for hospitalisation [54–56]. In contrast to the RECOVERY trial that takes place among hospitalised patients in the UK within a well-integrated health system with a national health insurance scheme, the TOGETHER trial is an outpatient trial with trial sites in the state of Minas Gerais in

Brazil [54, 56]. The TOGETHER trial consists of a network of investigators affiliated with academic institutions in Brazil, Canada, and the United States and partnership with contracted research organisations providing data management and analytical support. The TOGETHER trial began recruitment in June 2020 and has enrolled over 6,000 outpatients. At the time of writing, it currently has included 11 interventions, with 6 interventions having been completed for evaluation. This is a rare example of an adaptive randomised platform trial that has been conducted in a resource-limited setting with a more fragmented health system than previous clinical trials that have been described thus far.

Design and Methods

In the TOGETHER trial, patients presenting to an outpatient clinical setting with presumptive diagnosis of COVID-19 undergo a reverse transcriptase-polymerase chain reaction (RT-PCR) or a rapid antigen test to confirm a positive diagnosis [56]. Eligible patients are randomly assigned at an equal allocation ratio to one of the study arms that are active for recruitment. This is a placebo-controlled study that uses different placebos that match the administration and formulation of the experimental interventions being compared [56]. The primary endpoint of this trial includes a composite endpoint hospitalisation defined as either retention in a COVID-19 emergency setting or transfer to tertiary hospital due to COVID-19 up to 28 days post-random assignment. The pairwise comparison against the common concurrent control is used as the primary analysis based on the intention-to-treat principle.

This trial uses sequential designs and sample size re-assessment procedures under the Bayesian statistical framework. Throughout the pandemic, different assumptions for control event rates were used due to the rapidly changing course of the disease [55, 57–59]. For the latest results on fluvoxamine, the initial target sample size was 681 participants per arm [58]. This was planned assuming a control event rate of 15% and a relative risk reduction (RRR) of 37.5% set as a minimally clinical important difference (MCID) to achieve 80% statistical power with 0.05 two-sided type 1 error. Interim analyses for early stopping based on futility and superiority were both planned. The threshold for futility stopping was defined as having less than 40% posterior probability of superiority, defined by having an RRR greater than 0 (null), at the interim analysis. The threshold for superiority was defined at 97.6%.

Findings

As of today, there are six interventions that have completed their clinical evaluation. From the TOGETHER trial, several results have now been peer reviewed and published on HCQ and lopinavir/ritonavir [55], fluvoxamine [58], ivermectin [57], and metformin [59]. While lack of clinical efficacy was confirmed in HCQ, lopinavir/ritonavir, ivermectin, and metformin, fluvoxamine offers clinical benefit in reducing the need for hospitalisation among high-risk outpatients with an early diagnosis of COVID-19 [58]. While the TOGETHER trial started on 2 June 2020, fluvoxamine was added into the platform on 20 January 2021 [58].

Between 20 January and 5 August 2021, 741 patients were randomly assigned to fluvoxamine and 756 into the concurrent placebo control arm. In comparison to the placebo, the proportion of patients who were hospitalised was lower for the fluvoxamine group compared with placebo. Eleven per cent of patients assigned to fluvoxamine ($n = 79/741$) became hospitalised, whereas 16% of patients assigned to the control ($n = 119/756$) became hospitalised. Fluvoxamine had a 99.8% probability of superiority versus the placebo with a relative risk of 0.68 (95% CI: 0.52, 0.88) in terms of the composite hospitalisation endpoint. Fluvoxamine is an affordable therapeutic option at a current price of approximately $1 per day with decades of safety data and large manufacturing capacity at the global level [60]. This is one of the important milestones for COVID-19 that the investigators of the TOGETHER trial have been able to accomplish by establishing a resilient clinical trial infrastructure for pandemic research [54].

References

1. Park JJH, Siden E, Zoratti MJ, et al. Systematic review of basket trials, umbrella trials, and platform trials: a landscape analysis of master protocols. *Trials.* 2019;**20**(1):572.

2. Vanderbeek AM, Bliss JM, Yin Z, Yap C. Implementation of platform trials in the COVID-19 pandemic: a rapid review. *Contemp Clin Trials.* 2022;**112**:106625.

3. Parmar MK, Barthel FM, Sydes M, et al. Speeding up the evaluation of new agents in cancer. *J Natl Cancer Inst.* 2008;**100**(17):1204–14.

4. James ND, Sydes MR, Clarke NW, et al. Systemic therapy for advancing or metastatic prostate cancer (STAMPEDE): a multi-arm, multistage randomized controlled trial. *BJU Int.* 2009;**103**(4):464–9.

5. Sydes MR, Parmar MKB, James ND, et al. Issues in applying multi-arm multi-stage methodology to a clinical trial in prostate cancer: the MRC STAMPEDE trial. *Trials.* 2009;**10**:39.

6. National Library of Medicine. Systemic Therapy in Advancing or Metastatic Prostate Cancer: Evaluation of Drug Efficacy (STAMPEDE). ClinicalTrials.gov Identifier NCT00268476; 22 December 2005, last updated 13 April 2022. https://clinicaltrials.gov/ct2/show/NCT00268476

7. James ND, Sydes MR, Clarke NW, et al. Addition of docetaxel, zoledronic acid, or both to first-line long-term hormone therapy in prostate cancer (STAMPEDE): survival results from an adaptive, multiarm, multistage, platform randomised controlled trial. *Lancet.* 2016;**387**(10024):1163–77.

8. Mason MD, Clarke NW, James ND, et al. Adding celecoxib with or without zoledronic acid for hormone-naïve prostate cancer: long-term survival results from an adaptive, multiarm, multistage, platform, randomized controlled trial. *J Clin Oncol.* 2017;**35**(14):1530.

9. James ND, de Bono JS, Spears MR, et al. Abiraterone for Prostate cancer not previously treated with hormone therapy. *N Engl J Med.* 2017;**377**(4):338–51.

10. Parker CC, James ND, Brawley CD, et al. Radiotherapy to the primary tumour for newly diagnosed, metastatic prostate cancer (STAMPEDE): a randomised controlled phase 3 trial. *Lancet.* 2018;**392**(10162):2353–66.

11. Attard G, Murphy L, Clarke NW, et al. Abiraterone acetate and prednisolone with or without enzalutamide for high-risk non-metastatic prostate cancer: a meta-analysis of primary results from two randomised controlled phase 3 trials of the STAMPEDE platform protocol. *Lancet.* 2022;**399**(10323):447–60.

12. James ND, Spears MR, Clarke NW, et al. Failure-free survival and radiotherapy in patients with newly diagnosed nonmetastatic prostate cancer: data from patients in the control arm of the STAMPEDE trial. *JAMA Oncol.* 2016;**2**(3):348–57.

13. Redman MW, Allegra CJ. The master protocol concept. *Semin Oncol.* 2015;**42**(5):724–30.

14. Royston P, Parmar MK, Qian W. Novel designs for multi-arm clinical trials with survival outcomes with an application in ovarian cancer. *Stat Med.* 2003;**22**(14):2239–56.

15. Millen GC, Yap C. Adaptive trial designs: what are multiarm, multistage trials? *Arch Dis Child Educ Prac.* 2020;**105**(6):376–8.

16. Park JJH, Harari O, Dron L, et al. An overview of platform trials with a checklist for clinical readers. *J Clin Epidemiol.* 2020;**125**:1–8.

17. Angus DC, Alexander BM, Berry S, et al. Adaptive platform trials: definition, design, conduct and reporting considerations. *Nat Rev Drug Discov.* 2019;**18**(10):797–807.

18. Sydes MR, James ND, Mason MD, et al. Flexible trial design in practice – dropping and adding arms in STAMPEDE: a multi-arm multi-stage randomised controlled trial. *Trials.* 2011;**12**(suppl. 1).

19. Sydes MR, Parmar MKB, Mason MD, et al. Flexible trial design in practice – stopping arms for lack-of-benefit and adding

research arms mid-trial in STAMPEDE: a multi-arm multi-stage randomized controlled trial. *Trials*. 2012;**13**:168.

20. Sweeney CJ, Chen YH, Carducci M, et al. Chemohormonal therapy in metastatic hormone-sensitive prostate cancer. *N Engl J Med*. 2015;**373**(8):737–46.

21. Gravis G, Boher JM, Joly F, et al. Androgen deprivation therapy (ADT) plus docetaxel versus ADT alone in metastatic non castrate prostate cancer: impact of metastatic burden and long-term survival analysis of the randomized phase 3 GETUG-AFU15 trial. *Eur Urol*. 2016;**70** (2):256–62.

22. Vale CL, Burdett S, Rydzewska LHM, et al. Addition of docetaxel or bisphosphonates to standard of care in men with localised or metastatic, hormone-sensitive prostate cancer: a systematic review and meta-analyses of aggregate data. *Lancet Oncol*. 2016;**17**(2):243–56.

23. Park JJH, Detry MA, Murthy S, Guyatt G, Mills EJ. How to use and interpret the results of a platform trial: users' guide to the medical literature. *JAMA*. 2022;**327** (1):67–74.

24. Woodcock J, LaVange LM. Master protocols to study multiple therapies, multiple diseases, or both. *N Engl J Med*. 2017;**377**(1):62–70.

25. Park JW, Liu MC, Yee D, et al. Adaptive randomization of neratinib in early breast cancer. *N Engl J Med*. 2016;**375**(1):11–22.

26. Rugo HS, Olopade OI, DeMichele A, et al. Adaptive randomization of veliparib-carboplatin treatment in breast cancer. *N Engl J Med*. 2016;**375**(1):23–34.

27. Barker AD, Sigman CC, Kelloff GJ, et al. I-SPY 2: an adaptive breast cancer trial design in the setting of neoadjuvant chemotherapy. *Clin Pharmacol Ther*. 2009;**86**(1):97–100.

28. Mook S, Van't Veer LJ, Rutgers EJ, Piccart-Gebhart MJ, Cardoso F. Individualization of therapy using Mammaprint: from development to the MINDACT trial. *Cancer Genomics Proteomics*. 2007;**4** (3):147–55.

29. Cardoso F, Van't Veer L, Rutgers E, et al. Clinical application of the 70-gene profile: the MINDACT trial. *J Clin Oncol*. 2008;**26** (5):729–35.

30. National Library of Medicine. I-SPY TRIAL: Neoadjuvant and Personalized Adaptive Novel Agents to Treat Breast Cancer (I-SPY). ClinicalTrials.gov Identifier NCT01042379; 5 January 2010; last updated 10 June 2022. https://clinical trials.gov/ct2/show/NCT01042379.

31. Das S, Lo AW. Re-inventing drug development: a case study of the I-SPY 2 breast cancer clinical trials program. *Contemp Clin Trials*. 2017;**62**:168–74.

32. Chien AJ, Tripathy D, Albain KS, et al. MK-2206 and standard neoadjuvant chemotherapy improves response in patients with human epidermal growth factor receptor 2–positive and/or hormone receptor–negative breast cancers in the I-SPY 2 trial. *J Clin Oncol*. 2020;**38** (10):1059.

33. Nanda R, Liu MC, Yau C, et al. Effect of pembrolizumab plus neoadjuvant chemotherapy on pathologic complete response in women with early-stage breast cancer: an analysis of the ongoing phase 2 adaptively randomized I-SPY2 trial. *JAMA Oncol*. 2020;**6** (5):676–84.

34. Wise J, Coombes R. Covid-19: the inside story of the RECOVERY trial. *BMJ*. 2020;**370**:m2670.

35. The RECOVERY trial. 2020. www .recoverytrial.net/

36. Park JJ, Mogg R, Smith GE, et al. How COVID-19 has fundamentally changed clinical research in global health. *Lancet Glob Health*. 2021;**9**(5):e711–e20.

37. Park JJ, Ford N, Xavier D, et al. Randomised trials at the level of the individual. *Lancet Glob Health*. 2021;**9**(5): e691–e700.

38. Park JJ, Grais RF, Taljaard M, et al. Urgently seeking efficiency and sustainability of clinical trials in global health. *Lancet Glob Health*. 2021;**9**(5): e681–e90.

39. Narhi F, Moonesinghe SR, Shenkin SD, et al. Implementation of corticosteroids in treatment of COVID-19 in the ISARIC WHO Clinical Characterisation Protocol UK: prospective, cohort study. *Lancet Digit Health*. 2022;**4**(4):e220–e34.

40. Recovery Collaborative Group, Horby P, Lim WS, Emberson JR, et al. Dexamethasone in hospitalized patients with Covid-19. *N Engl J Med*. 2021;**384**(8):693–704.

41. RC Group, Horby P, Lim WS, Emberson JR, et al. Dexamethasone in hospitalized patients with Covid-19. *N Engl J Med*. 2021;**384**(8):693–704.

42. NIHR. Recruiting patients for clinical trials for COVID-19 Therapeutics; 2020. www.nihr.ac.uk/documents/news/recruiting-patients-for-clinical-trials-for-covid-therapeutics.pdf

43. The RECOVERY trial. No clinical benefit from use of hydroxychloroquine in hospitalised patients with COVID-19. 2020. https://www.recoverytrial.net/news/statement-from-the-chief-investigators-of-the-randomised-evaluation-of-covid-19-therapy-recovery-trial-on-hydroxychloroquine-5-june-2020-no-clinical-benefit-from-use-of-hydroxychloroquine-in-hospitalised-patients-with-covid-19#:~:text=The%20RECOVERY%20Trial%20has%20shown,research%20on%20more%20promising%20drugs.

44. Horby P, Lim WS, Emberson J, et al. Effect of dexamethasone in hospitalized patients with COVID-19: preliminary report. *medRxiv*. 2020:**2020**.06.22.20137273.

45. RC Group. Casirivimab and imdevimab in patients admitted to hospital with COVID-19 (RECOVERY): a randomised, controlled, open-label, platform trial. *Lancet*. 2022;**399**(10325):665–76.

46. RC Group. Aspirin in patients admitted to hospital with COVID-19 (RECOVERY): a randomised, controlled, open-label, platform trial. *Lancet*. 2022;**399**(10320):143–51.

47. RC Group. Colchicine in patients admitted to hospital with COVID-19 (RECOVERY): a randomised, controlled, open-label, platform trial. *Lancet Respir Med*. 2021;**9**(12):1419–26.

48. RC Group. Convalescent plasma in patients admitted to hospital with COVID-19 (RECOVERY): a randomised controlled, open-label, platform trial. *Lancet*. 2021;**397**(10289):2049–59.

49. RC Group. Tocilizumab in patients admitted to hospital with COVID-19 (RECOVERY): a randomised, controlled, open-label, platform trial. *Lancet*. 2021;**397**(10285):1637–45.

50. RC Group. Azithromycin in patients admitted to hospital with COVID-19 (RECOVERY): a randomised, controlled, open-label, platform trial. *Lancet*. 2021;**397**(10274):605–12.

51. RC Group. Lopinavir-ritonavir in patients admitted to hospital with COVID-19 (RECOVERY): a randomised, controlled, open-label, platform trial. *Lancet*. 2020;**396**(10259):1345–52.

52. RC Group, Horby P, Mafham M, et al. Effect of hydroxychloroquine in hospitalized patients with Covid-19. *N Engl J Med*. 2020;**383**(21):2030–40.

53. Park JJH, Dron L, Mills EJ. Moving forward in clinical research with master protocols. *Contemp Clin Trials*. 2021;**106**:106438.

54. Forrest JI, Rawat A, Duailibe F, et al. Resilient clinical trial infrastructure in response to the COVID-19 pandemic: lessons learned from the TOGETHER randomized platform clinical trial. *Am J Trop Med Hyg*. 2022;**106**(2):389–93.

55. Reis G, Moreira Silva EAdS, Medeiros Silva DC, et al. Effect of early treatment with hydroxychloroquine or lopinavir and ritonavir on risk of hospitalization among patients with COVID-19: the TOGETHER randomized clinical trial. *JAMA Netw Open*. 2021;**4**(4):e216468–e.

56. Reis G, Moreira Silva EAdS, Silva DCM, et al. A multi-center, adaptive, randomized, platform trial to evaluate the effect of repurposed medicines in outpatients with early coronavirus disease 2019 (COVID-19) and high-risk for complications: the TOGETHER master trial protocol. *Gates Open Res*. 2021;**5**:117.

57. Reis G, Silva E, Silva DCM, et al. Effect of early treatment with ivermectin among patients with Covid-19. *N Engl J Med*. 2022.

58. Reis G, Dos Santos Moreira-Silva EA, Silva DCM, et al. Effect of early treatment with fluvoxamine on risk of emergency care and hospitalisation among patients with COVID-19: the TOGETHER randomised, platform clinical trial. *Lancet Glob Health*. 2022;**10**(1):e42–e51.

59. Reis G, Silva EAdSM, Silva DCM, et al. Effect of early treatment with metformin on risk of emergency care and hospitalization among patients with COVID-19: the TOGETHER randomized platform clinical trial. *Lancet Regional Health-Americas*. 2022;**6**:100142.

60. Lee TC, Vigod S, Bortolussi-Courval E, et al. Fluvoxamine for outpatient management of COVID-19 to prevent hospitalization: a systematic review and meta-analysis. *JAMA Netw Open*. 2022;**5**(4):e226269.

Case Studies of Basket Trials and Umbrella Trials

Jay J. H. Park, Edward J. Mills, and J. Kyle Wathen

Introduction

Basket trials refer to clinical trials in which one or more targeted therapies are evaluated on multiple diseases that share common molecular alterations or risk factors that may help predict whether the patients will respond to the given therapy. Umbrella trials refer to clinical trials in which multiple targeted therapies are evaluated for a single disease that is stratified into multiple sub-studies based on their molecular or other predictive risk factors. As these designs follow the core principle of precision medicine that aims to tailor interventions based on their genetic or other risk factors, they have been mostly applied in the field of oncology. In this chapter, we review six case studies of basket and umbrella trials that either have already been conducted or that have been ongoing for several years.

Basket Trials

Case Study 11.1: Trial of Ado-Trastuzumab Emtansine for Patients with HER2 Amplified or Mutant Cancers

Background

Human epidermal growth factor receptor 2 (HER2) is an emerging target in multiple cancers [1]. As HER2 mutation is known to contribute to the development of cancer (an oncogene), there has been investigation of HER2 targeted therapies in cancers with HER2 mutations. Ado-trastuzumab emtansine is an anti-HER2 monoclonal antibody combined with a microtubular inhibitor that was approved for metastatic breast cancer by the U.S. Food and Drug Administration (FDA) in 2019 [2, 3]. Based on ado-trastuzumab emtansine's biological mechanistic pathway, Li and colleagues conducted a multi-histology basket trial to test ado-trastuzumab emtansine as a potential targeted therapy that can produce antitumour response in HER2 amplified or mutant cancers regardless of their histology [4]. In 2018, they published results based on their phase IIA basket trial that evaluated whether ado-trastuzumab emtansine could achieve anti-tumour response in HER2 amplified or mutant cancers of multiple histologies (NCT02675829) [4, 5].

Design and Methods

In this basket trial, Li et al. recruited advanced lung, endometrial, salivary gland, biliary tract, ovarian, bladder, colorectal, and other cancers with HER2 amplification or mutation as a common eligibility criterion in order to evaluate whether this HER2-targeting drug warrants further evaluation [5]. In other words, HER2 amplification or mutation was the common predictive biomarker risk factor that was hypothesised to predict whether cancer patients with different histological types would respond to ado-trastuzumab emtansine.

All patients received weight-based (i.e., 3.6 mg/kg) intravenous fusion of ado-trastuzumab emtansine every 21 days until disease progression or unacceptable toxicity. The primary endpoint was overall response rate (ORR) defined as having a complete response (CR) or a partial response (PR) based on an outcome assessment called Response Evaluation Criteria in Solid Tumours (RECIST) version 1.1. In brief, tumour response is determined based on the changes the tumour size after treatment administration in comparison to baseline [6]. In RECIST version 1.1, CR is defined by the disappearance of all target tumours; whereas PR is defined by a 30% or greater decrease in the sum of the longest diameter of the target lesions from baseline [6].

In general, the primary objective of a phase IIA trial is to determine whether the drug being studied has sufficient biological activity that warrants further clinical evaluation [7]. Most phase IIA trials in oncology are conducted as a single-arm, non-randomised design that aims to obtain an estimate of anti-tumour effect measured by tumour response. If the proportion of patients whose tumours shrink by at least 30% (i.e., ORR) is greater than some desirable level, it is generally considered that the agent has sufficient activity that warrants further clinical evaluation. For phase IIA trials in oncology, a two-stage design that allows for early futility stopping called a Simon's two-stage design is the most commonly used multi-stage design [7]. Simon two-stage design is also the most commonly used approach in basket trials, which the investigators of this multi-histology basket trial used as well [7, 8].

In Simon's two-stage design, a trial is conducted in two stages with the option to stop the trial after the first or the second stage depending on the response observed [7]. It aims to minimise the number of patients treated if the null hypothesis is true. The null hypothesis is defined using a true response rate that is considered to be either 'uninteresting' or 'undesirable'. The response rate under the null hypothesis could be considered as potentially dangerous for the patients being treated. The alternative hypothesis is defined with a desirable response rate that would warrant further investigation. Based on these pre-specified response rates, desired type I error rate, and power, Simon's two-stage design assumes an overall maximum number of patients (N), with a sub-set recruited for the first stage (n1). The trial is stopped early for futility if the minimum pre-specified tumour response is not observed at the first stage (r1). If the minimum response is observed, the trial continues recruitment up to N; at the second stage, the null hypothesis is rejected if the overall number of responders exceeds r. Simon's two-stage design may be designed to minimise the maximum sample size ('minimax design') or the expected sample size under the null hypothesis ('optimal design') [7].

In this multi-histology basket trial, they used the Simon's optimal design [4]. The trial set the target accrual for each cohort at a minimum of 7 patients for the first stage and 11 patients for the second stage for a maximum sample size of 18 patients [4]. This allowed for 89% statistical power at 2.7% one-sided type I error rate that considered a true ORR of 10% or less to be unacceptable (null hypothesis) and a minimum 40% ORR as desirable (alternative hypothesis) [4]. If there were no responses observed after the first stage, the trial would not continue into the second stage for that cohort. Controlling the type I error rate at 2.7% in each cohort meant that there was an overall master protocol-wise type I error rate of 10% [4]. In other words, there was at most 10% probability of making at least one type I error rate across all comparisons outlined in the master protocol.

Findings

For the cohort of HER2-mutant lung cancers, 18 eligible patients ended up being enrolled, meaning that the cohort in the first stage showed a sufficient number of responses [4]. The demonstrated ORR was 44% (95% CI: 22%, 69%). Eight out of 18 patients all had partial responses to the treatment, and there were no patients who had a complete response. An additional 39% of patients achieved stable disease, meaning the tumour did not grow any bigger, for up to 11 months. The investigators highlighted the promise of ado-trastuzumab emtansine as a targeted therapy for this molecular sub-set of lung cancers with HER2 mutation and recommended further evaluation of this agent.

Among HER2 amplified tumours, the investigators reported the results that included 53 patients across 8 cohorts of advanced lung, endometrial, salivary gland, biliary tract, ovarian, bladder, colorectal, and other cancers [5]. ORR was 26% ($n = 14/53$; 95% CI 15–40%). The ORR for HER2 amplified lung cancers was 50% ($n = 3/6$), 22% (4/18) for endometrial cancers, 100% (5/5) for salivary cancers, 17% (1/6) for biliary cancers, and 17% (1/6) for ovarian cancers.

Case Study 11.2: NCI-MATCH

Background

The Molecular Analysis for Therapy Choice (NCI-MATCH) of the National Cancer Institute (NCI) is a phase IIA basket trial for advanced refractory solid tumour, lymphoma, or multiple myeloma patients who have progressed on their previous treatment (NCT02465060) [9–12]. This trial is part of NCI's precision medicine initiative in the United States that aimed to study therapies targeting molecular biomarkers with low frequency (<10%) in solid tumours or lymphomas that have progressed following at least one line of standard treatment or for which no agreed upon treatment approach exists [13]. This is one of the largest biomarker-guided trials to date. It started in August 2015 with 10 treatment arms [14]. According to the U.S. National Library of Medicine ClinicalTrials.gov (NCT02465060), as of 22 April 2022, the trial has expanded to 1,425 sites actively recruiting patients of 50 different tumour types.

Design and Methods

NCI-MATCH is a non-randomised trial that assigns a specific targeted therapy for each of the molecular sub-types regardless of their histological tumour type [12]. As part of its master protocol, patients undergo a mandatory biopsy whereby a sample of tumour tissue is obtained for a centralised molecular screening using next generation sequencing assay for detection of actionable mutations of interest [12]. Then patients would be assigned to the sub-protocol that is defined by their molecular sub-type. There are 38 treatment sub-protocols that are determined based on their molecular sub-type. All patients are followed up every three months for two years, then every six months for one year after the completion of their assigned targeted therapy.

It uses a single-stage design with an accrual goal of 35 patients to obtain 31 eligible patients for each molecular group assuming 10% of the enrolled patients would later be deemed ineligible [15, 16]. An ORR of 16% or larger ($n \geq 5/31$) was considered to be promising and worthy of further testing [12]. Enrolling 31 patients would have 91.8% power to conclude that an agent is promising assuming a true response rate of 25%, and 1.8% one-sided type I error rate if the true response rate is 5% [15, 16].

Findings

For this chapter, we focus on results out of the NCI-MATCH's sub-protocol W that included patients with tumours harbouring fibroblast growth factor receptor (FGFR) 1–3 who were treated with an oral FGFR1–3 inhibitor, AZD4547 [15]. Between July 2016 and June 2017, of the 70 patients who assigned to sub-protocol W, 48 (69%) received the assigned therapy and were eligible for statistical analysis [15]. After the initial accrual of 35 patients, the protocol was expanded to accrue up to 70 patients based on the new findings that AZD4547 did not show promising anti-tumour activity in lung cancers, gastric cancers, or gastroesophageal junction cancers with FGFR1–3 amplification [17–19]. The ORR was 8% ($n = 4/48$; 95% CI: 3%, 18%). Out of these 48 patients, there were 20 patients with FGFR1 or 2 amplification, 19 with FGFR2 or 3 single nucleotide variant (SNV) mutation, and 9 with FGFR1 and 3 fusion [15]. Patients with FGFR1 and 3 fusion did show a higher ORR of 22% ($n = 2/9$). However, this was based on a small number of patients, and the trial was not powered to detect a sub-group effect among different types of FGFR1–3 mutations. While the finding on AZD4547 as a targeted therapy for FGFR 1–3 mutation is negative, the trial has tested and continues to test other therapies as potential targeted therapies for different mutations.

Case Study 11.3: NCI-MPACT

Background

The NCI's Molecular Profiling-Based Assignment of Cancer Therapy (NCI-MPACT) is another basket trial that aims to test tumour-agnostic approaches in targeted treatment selection [20, 21]. In contrast to case study 2 (NCI-MATCH), this trial is a randomised clinical trial with eight sites recruiting patients with advanced refractory solid tumours [22]. This trial is testing the efficacy of applying tumour DNA sequencing to treatment selection as an intervention versus an approach that would not use such information as a targeted therapy. In this basket trial, 20 genes belonging to three pathways of RAS/RAF/MEK (five genes), PI3K/mTOR/AKT (five genes), and DNA repair (ten genes) are being evaluated as treatment selection approaches of four potential targeted therapies [20, 21].

There are four regimens being evaluated: (1) trametinib (MEK inhibitor); (2) everolimus (mTOR inhibitor); (3) veliparib (PARP inhibitor) + temozolomide (TMZ; alkylating agent); and (4) adavosertib (tyrosine kinase WEE1 inhibitor) + carboplatin. Trametinib is being evaluated as a targeted therapy for the RAS pathway. Everolimus being evaluated for the PI3K pathway, and two regimens of veliparib + TMZ and adavosertib + carboplatin are being evaluated for the DNA repair pathway [22].

Design and Methods

NCI-MPACT is a two-arm randomised clinical trial in which patients were randomly assigned to one of the four regimens being used as a targeted therapy based on their genetic mutations (experimental arm: targeted therapy group) or to one of the same four regimens but chosen not based on their genetic mutations (control arm: non-targeted therapy group) [23].

Patients harbouring the corresponding genetic mutations were randomised 2:1 into the targeted therapy group or into the control group [22]. For each regimen cohort of the experimental arm, up to 30 patients could be recruited to discriminate between tumour response rates of 20% versus 5% [23]. Two-stage design was used for tumour response assessment. If no objective responses (PR or CR) were observed in the initial 12 patients in each mutation sub-category, the cohort was terminated early for futility [23]. At the end of the second (final) stage, the regimen would have been considered promising for the specific mutation sub-category if at least four objective responses (ORR of 13% or greater) would have been observed [23].

For the randomised trial design aspect, the total target recruitment was 180 evaluable patients (120 to experimental intervention and 60 to control) for 88% statistical power at 4% one-sided type I error rate to detect an overall difference of 20% versus 5% for objective response outcome and 90% statistical power and 1% one-sided type I error rate for an 80% increase in median progression-free survival [22].

Findings

Between 2014 and 2018, 64 patients were randomly assigned to the treatment group and 32 patients were assigned to the control group for a total of 96 patients who had a target mutation [23]. Of the 64 patients assigned to the treatment group, 49 received the assigned therapy, and 16 out of 32 patients randomly assigned to the control group ended up being treated. The ORRs in both groups were low. The ORR in the treatment group was 2% ($n = 1/49$; 95% CI: 0%, 10.9%) and 0% for the control group [23]. Within the treatment group, 20 out of 25 patients assigned to trametinib received the assigned therapy in the first regimen. Only 1 of 20 patients (5%) had a PR, so this was decided not to be a promising targeted therapy for the patients harbouring RAS mutations. The second (everolimus; $n = 8$) and third (veliparib + TMZ; $n = 3$) regimens of the treatment groups did not meet the accrual target, and no responses were observed in these cohort regimens [23]. Accrual to the fourth regimen, adavosertib + carboplatin, was met, but there were no confirmed responses ($n = 0/18$), indicating statistical futility [23].

The challenges associated with conducting biomarker-guided randomised clinical trials in an advanced disease settings are highlighted from this case study. Both patients and physicians were blinded to the sequencing and random assignment results, but a higher pre-treatment dropout rate has been reported for the control arm (22%; $n = 7/32$) in comparison to the experimental arm (6%; $n = 4/64$) [23]. According to the trial investigators of NCI-MPACT, there is preference for targeted therapies that make it difficult to evaluate such strategies using a randomised clinical trial design [23]. Despite having a 90% successful biopsy collection rate with a turnaround time of 10 days or less for genomic sequencing results, the trial did not meet recruitment targets in two of four experimental regimens due to low prevalence of the targeted mutations [23].

Umbrella Trials

Case Study 11.4: plasmaMATCH

Background

The plasmaMATCH trial (NCT03182634) is an umbrella trial that evaluated five different therapies for advanced breast cancer [24–27]. This trial used a blood test (plasma test) to detect circulating tumour DNA (ctDNA) on targeted genetic mutations to decide treatments for advanced breast cancer. ctDNA is found in the plasma of over 90% of patients with advanced breast cancer, and thus ctDNA screening could be used as a targeted treatment strategy [26, 27].

Design and Methods

The plasmaMATCH trial was a phase IIA, non-randomised clinical trial using a plasma test for circulating tumour DNA in blood. Patients were assigned to one of the targeted therapies based on their genetic mutation. In this umbrella trial, multiple biomarker assays were applied to a single tumour histology, and patients were assigned to one of the five groups based on their biomarker status to evaluate the clinical utility of five different targeted therapy strategies for advanced breast cancer. The therapies were stratified as five treatment groups based on their molecular signatures These five breast cancer groups were as follows:

1) Group A: *ESR1* mutation (oestrogen receptor gene 1)
2) Group B: *HER2* mutation (human epidermal growth factor receptor 2)
3) Group C: *AKT* mutation (a serine/threonine-specific protein kinase B)
4) Group D: *AKT* activation
5) Group E: Triple negative (*ESR1, HER2,* and *AKT* negative) status

Patients with *ESR1* mutation in Group A received an extended dose of an oestrogen receptor down regulator, fulvestrant (500 mg every two weeks) [24, 25, 28]. Patients with *HER2* mutation in Group B received an HER tyrosine kinase inhibitor in neratinib and additionally fulvestrant if they had an oestrogen receptor co-mutation [24, 25, 29]. Patients with *AKT* mutation in Group C received an *AKT* inhibitor in AZD5364 plus fulvestrant, whereas patients with *AKT* activation in Group D received AZD5364 only [25]. Lastly, for Group E, patients with triple negative breast cancer received a poly(ADP-ribose)polymerase (PARP) inhibitor in olaparib plus AZD5364 [24, 25, 30].

All groups used a single-stage design that aimed for 80% statistical power at 5% two-sided type I error rate for each group [27]. The recruitment target for Group A was 78 evaluable patients to infer tumour activity and required 13 or more objective tumour responses for the agent to be considered promising. This was determined based on a 20% target response rate and a 10% response rate to be unacceptable. For Groups B, C, and D each assumed a target response rate of 25% and a 5% response rate was unacceptable. The regimen was considered to be promising and warrant further clinical investigation if it demonstrated three or more responses from 16 evaluable patients.

Findings

Between December 2016 and April 2019, a total of 1,051 patients were registered into this trial [27]. Of these patients, 1,044 (99%) underwent ctDNA testing. Thirty-four per cent ($n = 357/1,044$) of these patients had target mutations, and a total of 136 patients were assigned to the different groups [27]. In Group A with ESR1 mutation, 80 out of 84 patients received fulvestrant, and 74 were evaluated for tumour response. In Group B with HER2 mutation, 20 out of 21 patients received neratinib +/– fulvestrant and evaluated for tumour response. Eighteen patients with AKT mutation entered Group C and received AZD5364 + fulvestrant; 19 patients with AKT activation entered Group D and received AZD5364 only. There was only one triple-negative breast cancer patient who entered Group E.

In Group A that had 13 or more tumour responses as a target, only 6 out of 74 patients had an objective response (ORR of 8%; 95% CI: 3%, 17%) [27]. In Groups B, C, and D, the target number of responses was three or more. Group B and Group C exceeded the target number of responses, whereas Group D did not. Five out of 20 patients in Group B had an objective response (ORR: 25%; 95% CI: 9%, 49%), and 4 out of 18 patients in Group C had an objective response (ORR: 22%; 95% CI: 6%, 48%). In Group D, only 2 out of 19 patients had an objective response (ORR of 11%; 95% CI: 1%, 33%) [27].

Case Study 11.5: ALCHEMIST Trial

Background

Adjuvant Lung Cancer Enrichment Marker Identification and Sequencing Trial (ALCHEMIST) is an umbrella trial that started in August 2014 for patients with operable early stage (IB–IIIA) lung adenocarcinoma, a common histological sub-type of non-squamous non-small cell lung cancer (NSCLC) [31]. ALCHEMIST is evaluating targeted therapies based on two genetic mutations that are believed to be important for lung cancer: EGFR and ALK mutations.

Design and Methods

There are multiple sub-protocols of ALCHEMIST:
 1) ALCHEMIST Screening (A151216; NCT02194738);
 2) ALCHEMIST-EGFR (A081105; NCT02193282);
 3) ALCHEMIST-ALK sub-protocol (E4512; NCT02201992);
 4) ALCHEMIST-Immunotherapy Treatment Trial (ANVIL: EA5142; NCT02595944); and
 5) ALCHEMIST Chemo-IO study (A081801; NCT04267848).

The ALCHEMIST Screening study has been established for centralised screening of adenocarcinoma patients across the United States for a genomic analysis of EGFR mutations and ALK rearrangement [32]. The ALCHEMIST Screening study will screen up to 8,000 adeno-carcinoma patients before or after surgical resection, and based on their genomic analysis, they will be assigned to other ALCHEMIST sub-protocols. Patients with EGFR mutation are assigned to the ALCHEMIST-EGFR sub-protocol for an assessment of the clinical efficacy of an EGFR inhibitor called erlotinib [33]. Patients with ALK rearrangement are assigned to the ALCHEMIST-ALK sub-protocol for an assessment of an ALK and ROS1 inhibitor, crizotinib [33]. Lastly, patients who do not have EGFR or ALK mutations, regardless of their PD-L1 expression level, will be assigned to the fourth sub-protocol ANVIL studying nivolumab (PD-L1 inhibitor) [33].

ALCHEMIST-EGFR, ALCHEMIST-ALK, and ANVIL are phase 3 randomised clinical trials with the primary endpoint of overall survival (OS). ALCHEMIST-EGFR is a placebo-controlled randomised clinical trial evaluating erlotinib. This trial uses a fixed trial design with equal allocation ratio and the final statistical analysis taking place once 183 deaths are observed [31]. The target accrual is 410 patients that will allow for an 85% power at 5% one-sided type I error rate to detect a 33% reduction in OS hazard rate (a hazard ratio of 0.67) favour of the treatment using a log-rank test. It assumed a median OS of 60 months in the control group. ALCHEMIST-ALK is another placebo-controlled randomised clinical trial evaluating crizotinib [31]. It has an enrolment target of 360 patients (180 patients per arm) with a targeted overall number of events of 164 [31]. The trial will have 80% power at 5% one-sided type I error rate to detect a hazard ratio of 0.67 using a log-rank test assuming a median OS of 66 months in the placebo group. Assuming an exponent survival distribution, a hazard ratio of 0.67 would translate to a 50% improvement in median duration of OS in the treated group. ANVIL will use a standard observational arm as the control and will recruit 714 patients to detect a 30% improvement in OS and/or 33% reduction in disease-free survival favouring nivolumab [33].

It has been reported that ALCHEMIST has added a new sub-study called ALCHEMIST Chemo-IO study (A081801; NCT04267848) in June 2020 [34]. Patients in this sub-study will be randomly assigned to one of three arms: (1) chemo-IO with pembrolizumab during and after chemo; (2) sequential chemo followed by pembrolizumab; and (3) chemo alone. The specific design features, such as sample size calculations, for this sub-study have not been reported.

Findings

To the best of our knowledge, there has not been any read-outs from ALCHEMIST-EGFR, ALCHEMIST-ALK, nor ANVIL. There is a readout from the ALCHEMIST Screening study in May 2020 [34] and March 2022 [32]. Between August 2014 and January 2020, there have been 5,362 patients who were registered into the screening study [34]. There have been 352 patients randomised in the ALCHEMIST-EGFR study, 99 patients in the ALCHEMIST-ALK study, and 935 patients in the ANVIL study. While early progress is not reported for the ALCHEMIST Chemo-IO study, it is encouraging that the ALCHEMIST platform is being used to another research question within their trial network.

Case Study 11.6: Lung-MAP

Background

The Lung Cancer Master Protocol (Lung-Map) is one of the largest umbrella trials has been ongoing since June 2014. Lung-MAP started recruiting patients with advanced squamous non-small cell lung cancer (NSCLC) into five sub-studies (S1400A-E; NCT02154490) [35]. Over time, Lung-MAP has added two more non-match sub-studies (S1400F and S1400I) and two other biomarker-driven sub-studies (S1400G and S1400 K) for squamous NSCLC patients. On 28 January 2019, Lung-Map was expanded to all histological types of NSCLC under a new screening protocol, S1900 (NCT03851445), that aims to test other targeted and non-targeted therapies under one single master protocol [36]. It currently has over 800 trial sites across the United States.

Design and Methods

Lung-MAP is an umbrella trial that has established centralised genomic screening for simultaneous accrual into multiple sub-studies based on patients' genetic mutations. There are both non-randomised and randomised sub-studies that have operated under the Lung-MAP master protocol. Lung-MAP originally started with five sub-studies, S1400A to S1400E [35, 37]. The first sub-study (S1400A) was a single-arm, non-match study, whereas the other four sub-studies, S1400B to S14000E, were biomarker-driven and investigated targeted therapies with two-arm seamless phase II/III randomised clinical trial designs [35, 37]. In S1400A, patients with tumours that did not have actionable molecular alterations that were used to assign patients into other biomarker-driven sub-studies were assigned into S1400A and received durvalumab, an anti-PDL1 monoclonal antibody [37]. Sub-study S1400B investigated a PI3K inhibitor, taselisib, in patients with a PIK3CA mutation [38]. Sub-study S1400C investigated a selective CDK4/6 inhibitor, palbociclib, in patients with CDK4, CCND1, CCND2, or CCND3 amplification [39], and S1400D investigated AZD4547 (an FGFR inhibitor) among patients with FGFR1, 2, or 3 mutation, fusion, or amplification [35]. These three sub-studies used docetaxel as the control [35]. The fifth sub-study, S1400E, was designed to investigate rilotumumab versus erlotinib for patients with MET mutation, but it closed due to a withdrawal from the manufacturer who observed toxicity of rilotumumab from other independent phase III trials [35]. As shown in Table 10.1, there have been multiple other sub-studies that have been added into the Lung-MAP trial infrastructure since then. As each sub-study had different design features, they will not be discussed individually here.

Findings

To the best of our knowledge, while the results of S1900 and S1800 sub-studies have not been published, several S1400 sub-studies of Lung-MAP have been published [18, 40–46]. It is not practical to report on all results due to the high number of sub-studies that have been published, so we will discuss Lung-MAP broadly.

Lung-MAP was created to establish a common infrastructure for biomarker screening and evaluation of multiple targeted therapies with an intention of their being considered for regulatory approval [48]. Across S1400 sub-studies, 1,864 patients with squamous NSCLC who were enrolled between June 2014 and January 2019 when S1400 protocols were closed in Lung-MAP [48]. Of these, 99% (n =1,841/1,864) submitted their tissue for biomarker screening, and 91% (n = 1,674/1,841) received their biomarker results [48]. Eighty-four per cent of patients (n = 1,404/1,674) with biomarker results received a sub-study assignment, and 47% of patients (n = 655/1,404) ended up being enrolled [48]. This was the first chapter of Lung-MAP, and it is continuing with a broader scope that includes all histological types of NSCLC and new therapies that had not been pre-specified before.

Lung-MAP is a classic example of an umbrella trial. It remains unclear whether there is a consensus to describe Lung-MAP as being a platform trial since new interventions have been added into the platform. This might be a discussion for semantics, but it is clear that Lung-MAP is a huge accomplishment for the cancer community. Lung-MAP has been made possible through a public–private partnership including the Cancer Therapy Evaluation Program (CTEP) at the NCI, the adult NCTN groups (Alliance for Clinical Trials in Oncology, Eastern Cooperative Oncology Group – American College of Radiology Imaging Network [ECOG-ACRIN], NRG Oncology, and SWOG Cancer Research Network), the Foundation for the National Institutes of Health, and Friends of Cancer Research.

Table 11.1 Lung-MAP sub-studies

Protocol	Target mutation	Therapy
Squamous cell non-small cell lung cancer		
S1400A [40]	–	Durvalumab (ipilimumab naïve)
S1400B [41]	Pi3 K+	Taselisib
S1400C [42]	CCGA+	Palbociclib
S1400D [18]	FGFR+	AZD4547
S1400E	c–MET+	Rilotumumab + erlotinib
S1400F [43]	–	Durvalumab + tremelimumab (Ipilimumab refractory)
S1400G [44]	HRRD+	Talazoparib
S1400I [45]	–	Nivolumab + ipilimumab (Ipilimumab naïve)
S1400 K [46]	c–MET+	Teliso-V (ABBV-399)
S1400 GEN [47]– A screening protocol (NCT03851445)[*]		
All histological types of non-small cell lung cancer (NCT03851445)		
S1900A	LOH/BRCA+	Rucaparib
S1900B	RET fus+	Selpercatinib (LOXO-292)
S1900C	STK11+	Talazoparib + avelumab
S1900D	NFE2L2 KEAP1+	TAK228 + docetaxel
S1900E	KRASG12C	Sotorasib
S1900F	RET fusion +	Selpercatinib + carboplatin + pemetrexed
S1800A	–	Pembrolizumab + ramucirumab (ipilimumab refractory)
S1800B	PI3 K+	Taselisib (sub-study on squamous lung cancer)
S1800C	–	Entionstat + pembrolizumab
S1800D	–	N-803 [ALT-803] + pembrolizumab
S1900 – A screening protocol (NCT03851445)[**]		

[*] S1400 GEN is a screening protocol for S1400 sub-studies of Lung-MAP.
[**] S1900 refers to a modified screening protocol that was adopted when Lung-MAP was expanded to include non-squamous lung cancer.

References

1. Connell CM, Doherty GJ. Activating HER2 mutations as emerging targets in multiple solid cancers. *ESMO Open.* 2017;2(5): e000279.

2. Verma S, Miles D, Gianni L, et al. Trastuzumab emtansine for HER2-positive advanced breast cancer. *N Engl J Med.* 2012;367(19):1783–91.

3. Amiri-Kordestani L, Blumenthal GM, Xu QC, et al. FDA approval: ado-trastuzumab emtansine for the treatment of patients with HER2-positive

metastatic breast cancer. *Clin Cancer Res.* 2014;**20**(17):4436–41.

4. Li BT, Shen R, Buonocore D, et al. Ado-trastuzumab emtansine for patients with HER2-mutant lung cancers: results from a phase II basket trial. *J Clin Oncol.* 2018;**36** (24):2532–7.

5. Li BT, Makker V, Buonocore DJ, et al. A multi-histology basket trial of ado-trastuzumab emtansine in patients with HER2 amplified cancers. *J Clin Oncol.* 2018;**36**(15_suppl):2502.

6. Eisenhauer EA, Therasse P, Bogaerts J, et al. New response evaluation criteria in solid tumours: revised RECIST guideline (version 1.1). *Eur J Cancer.* 2009;**45** (2):228–47.

7. Simon R. Optimal two-stage designs for phase II clinical trials. *Control Clin Trials.* 1989;**10**(1):1–10.

8. Park JJ, Harari O, Dron L, Mills EJ, Thorlund K. Effects of biomarker diagnostic accuracy on biomarker-guided phase 2 trials. *Contemp Clin Trials Commun.* 2019;**15**:100396.

9. Conley BA, Doroshow JH. Molecular analysis for therapy choice: NCI MATCH. *Semin Oncol.* 2014;**41**(3):297–9.

10. Mullard A. NCI-MATCH trial pushes cancer umbrella trial paradigm. *Nat Rev Drug Discov.* 2015;**14**(8):513–5.

11. Chen A, Conley B, Hamilton S, et al. NCI-Molecular Analysis for Therapy Choice (NCI-MATCH) trial: a novel public-private partnership. *Eur J Cancer.* 2016;**69**:S137.

12. Moore KN, Mannel RS. Is the NCI MATCH trial a match for gynecologic oncology? *Gynecol Oncol.* 2016;**140**(1):161–6.

13. Abrams J, Conley B, Mooney M, et al. National Cancer Institute's Precision Medicine Initiatives for the new National Clinical Trials Network. *Am Soc Clin Oncol Educ Book.* 2014:71–6.

14. Barroilhet L, Matulonis U. The NCI-MATCH trial and precision medicine in gynecologic cancers. *Gynecol Oncol.* 2018;**148**(3):585–90.

15. Chae YK, Hong F, Vaklavas C, et al. Phase II study of AZD4547 in patients with

tumors harboring aberrations in the FGFR pathway: results from the NCI-MATCH trial (EAY131) subprotocol W. *J Clin Oncol.* 2020;**38**(21):2407–17.

16. Mansfield AS, Wei Z, Mehra R, et al. Crizotinib in patients with tumors harboring ALK or ROS1 rearrangements in the NCI-MATCH trial. *NPJ Precis Oncol.* 2022;**6**(1):13.

17. Van Cutsem E, Bang YJ, Mansoor W, et al. A randomized, open-label study of the efficacy and safety of AZD4547 monotherapy versus paclitaxel for the treatment of advanced gastric adenocarcinoma with FGFR2 polysomy or gene amplification. *Ann Oncol.* 2017;**28** (6):1316–24.

18. Aggarwal C, Redman MW, Lara PN, Jr., et al. SWOG S1400D (NCT02965378), a phase II study of the fibroblast growth factor receptor inhibitor AZD4547 in previously treated patients with fibroblast growth factor pathway-activated stage IV squamous cell lung cancer (Lung-MAP Substudy). *J Thorac Oncol.* 2019;**14** (10):1847–52.

19. Aggarwal C, Redman MW, Lara P, et al. Phase II study of the FGFR inhibitor AZD4547 in previously treated patients with FGF pathway-activated stage IV squamous cell lung cancer (SqNSCLC): LUNG-MAP sub-study SWOG S1400D. *J Clin Oncol.* 2017;**35**(15 suppl).

20. Aggarwal C, Redman MW, Lara PN, Jr et al. SWOG S1400D (NCT02965378), a phase II study of the fibroblast growth factor receptor inhibitor AZD4547 in previously treated patients with fibroblast growth factor pathway–activated stage IV squamous cell lung cancer (Lung-MAP substudy). *J Thorac Oncol.* 2010;**14** (10):1847–1852.

21. Lih CJ, Takebe N. Considerations of developing an NGS assay for clinical applications in precision oncology: The NCI-MATCH NGS assay experience. *Curr Probl Cancer.* 2017;**41**(3):201–11.

22. Kummar S, Williams M, Lih C-J, et al. NCI mpact: National Cancer Institute molecular profiling-based assignment of cancer therapy. *J Clin Oncol.* 2014;**32**(15).

23. Chen AP, Kummar S, Moore N, et al. Molecular Profiling-Based Assignment of Cancer Therapy (NCI-MPACT): a randomized multicenter phase II trial. *JCO Precis Oncol.* 2021;5.

24. Turner N, Bye H, Kernaghan S, et al. Abstract OT1-06-03: The plasmaMATCH trial: A multiple parallel cohort, open-label, multi-centre phase II clinical trial of ctDNA screening to direct targeted therapies in patients with advanced breast cancer (CRUK/15/010). *Cancer Res.* 2018;78 (4 Supplement):OT1-06-3-OT1-3.

25. Cancer Research UK. A trial using a blood test to find certain gene changes and decide treatment for advanced breast cancer (plasmaMATCH). 2019. www .cancerresearchuk.org/about-cancer/ find-a-clinical-trial/a-trial-using-a-blood-test-to-find-certain-gene-changes-and-decide-treatment-for-advanced-breast#undefined

26. Kingston B, Cutts RJ, Bye H, et al. Genomic profile of advanced breast cancer in circulating tumour DNA. *Nat Commun.* 2021;12(1):2423.

27. Turner NC, Kingston B, Kilburn LS, et al. Circulating tumour DNA analysis to direct therapy in advanced breast cancer (plasmaMATCH): a multicentre, multicohort, phase 2a, platform trial. *Lancet Oncol.* 2020;21(10):1296–308.

28. Covens AL, Filiaci V, Gersell D, et al. Phase II study of fulvestrant in recurrent/ metastatic endometrial carcinoma: a Gynecologic Oncology Group study. *Gynecol Oncol.* 2011;120(2):185–8.

29. Rabindran SK, Discafani CM, Rosfjord EC, et al. Antitumor activity of HKI-272, an orally active, irreversible inhibitor of the HER-2 tyrosine kinase. *Cancer Res.* 2004;64 (11):3958–65.

30. Fong PC, Boss DS, Yap TA, et al. Inhibition of poly(ADP-ribose) polymerase in tumors from BRCA mutation carriers. *N Engl J Med.* 2009;361(2):123–34.

31. Govindan R, Mandrekar SJ, Gerber DE, Ox, et al. ALCHEMIST trials: a golden opportunity to transform outcomes in early-stage non-small cell lung cancer. *Clin Cancer Res.* 2015;21(24):5439–44.

32. Kehl KL, Zahrieh D, Yang P, et al. Rates of guideline-concordant surgery and adjuvant chemotherapy among patients with early-stage lung cancer in the US ALCHEMIST study (Alliance A151216). *JAMA Oncol.* 2022;8(5):717–28.

33. Chaft JE, Dahlberg SE, Khullar OV, et al. EA5142 adjuvant nivolumab in resected lung cancers (ANVIL). *J Clin Oncol.* 2018;35(15).

34. Sands J, Mandrekar SJ, Oxnard GR, K, et al. ALCHEMIST: Adjuvant targeted therapy or immunotherapy for high-risk resected NSCLC. *J Clin Oncol.* 2020;28 (15 suppl).

35. Ferrarotto R, Redman MW, Gandara DR, Herbst RS, Papadimitrakopoulou VA. Lung-MAP – framework, overview, and design principles. *Chin Clin Oncol.* 2015;4(3):36.

36. SWOG Cancer Research Network. A Master Protocol to Evaluate Biomarker-Driven Therapies and Immunotherapies in Previously-Treated Non-Small Cell Lung Cancer (Lung-MAP Screening Study). 2019. www.swog.org/clinical-trials/ lungmap

37. Papadimitrakopoulou V, Redman M, Borghaei H, et al. 83OA phase II study of durvalumab (MEDI4736) for previously treated patients with stage IV squamous NSCLC (SqNSCLC): Lung-MAP Sub-study SWOG S1400A. *Ann Oncol.* 2017;28 (suppl_2).

38. Wade JL, Langer CJ, Redman M, et al. A phase II study of GDC-0032 (taselisib) for previously treated PI3 K positive patients with stage IV squamous cell lung cancer (SqNSCLC): LUNG-MAP sub-study SWOG S1400B. *J Clin Oncol.* 2017;35(15).

39. Edelman MJ, Redman MW, Albain KS, et al. A phase II study of palbociclib (P) for previously treated cell cycle gene alteration positive patients (pts) with stage IV squamous cell lung cancer (SCC): Lung-MAP sub-study SWOG S1400C. *J Clin Oncol.* 2017;35(15).

40. Borghaei H, Redman MW, Kelly K, et al. SWOG S1400A (NCT02154490): a phase II study of durvalumab for patients with previously treated stage IV or recurrent squamous cell lung cancer (Lung-MAP sub-study). *Clin Lung Cancer.* 2021;**22** (3):178–86.

41. Langer CJ, Redman MW, Wade JL, 3rd, et al. SWOG S1400B (NCT02785913), a phase ii study of GDC-0032 (taselisib) for previously treated PI3 K-positive patients with stage IV squamous cell lung cancer (Lung-MAP sub-study). *J Thorac Oncol.* 2019;**14**(10):1839–46.

42. Edelman MJ, Redman MW, Albain KS, et al. SWOG S1400C (NCT02154490) – a phase II study of palbociclib for previously treated cell cycle gene alteration-positive patients with stage IV squamous cell lung cancer (Lung-MAP substudy). *J Thorac Oncol.* 2019;**14**(10):1853–9.

43. Leighl NB, Redman MW, Rizvi N, et al. Phase II study of durvalumab plus tremelimumab as therapy for patients with previously treated anti-PD-1/PD-L1 resistant stage IV squamous cell lung cancer (Lung-MAP substudy S1400F, NCT03373760). *J Immunother Cancer.* 2021;**9**(8).

44. Owonikoko TK, Redman MW, Byers LA, et al. Phase 2 study of talazoparib in patients with homologous recombination repair-deficient squamous cell lung cancer: Lung-MAP substudy S1400G. *Clin Lung Cancer.* 2021;**22** (3):187–94 e1.

45. Gettinger SN, Redman MW, Bazhenova L, et al. Nivolumab plus ipilimumab vs nivolumab for previously treated patients with stage IV squamous cell lung cancer: the Lung-MAP S1400I phase 3 randomized clinical trial. *JAMA Oncol.* 2021;**7** (9):1368–77.

46. Waqar SN, Redman MW, Arnold SM, et al. A phase II study of telisotuzumab vedotin in patients with c-MET-positive stage IV or recurrent squamous cell lung cancer (LUNG-MAP Sub-study S1400 K, NCT03574753). *Clin Lung Cancer.* 2021;**22** (3):170–7.

47. Roth JA, Trivedi MS, Gray SW, et al. Patient knowledge and expectations about return of genomic results in a biomarker-driven master protocol trial (SWOG S1400GEN). *JCO Oncology Pract.* 2021;**17**(11):e1821–e9.

48. Redman MW, Papadimitrakopoulou VA, Minichiello K, et al. Biomarker-driven therapies for previously treated squamous non-small-cell lung cancer (Lung-MAP SWOG S1400): a biomarker-driven master protocol. *Lancet Oncol.* 2020;**21** (12):1589–601.

12 Standards and Guidelines for Adaptive Trial Designs and Master Protocols

Jay J. H. Park, J. Kyle Wathen, and Edward J. Mills

Key Points of This Chapter

In this chapter, we discuss the standards and guidelines for adaptive trial designs and master protocols. The key points of this chapter are:

- Methodological rigour and transparent reporting are required in all clinical trials. Adaptive trial designs and master protocols are no exception. The standard reporting guidelines and risk-of-bias assessments for conventional trials can be applied to adaptive trial designs and master protocols.
- Adaptive trial designs have pre-planned adaptations and analysis plans that are specified in a formal way to outline how the data will be used to guide the design.
- Planning of adaptive clinical trials, basket trials, umbrella trials, and platform trials will require early engagement with the stakeholders and methodologists to think through potential hurdles and challenges of the statistical design and its implementation.

Introduction

Clinical trials are an important methodological tool to inform evidence-based medicine and public health policies [1]. By many, randomised clinical trials are considered the highest valid method for establishing efficacy of interventions [1]. It is imperative that clinical trials are designed and conducted with methodological rigour and reported with full transparency. To promote higher quality clinical trial research, standards for conventional clinical trials have generally been well established, evident by the several reporting guidelines and risk-of-bias assessment tools available. Most notably, there are the 'Standard Protocol Items: Recommendations for Interventional Trials' (SPIRIT) 2013 statement for complete documentation of clinical trial protocols [2], and the 'Consolidated Standards Of Reporting Trials' (CONSORT) 2010 statement for standard reporting items that should be included for randomised clinical trials [3, 4]. The Cochrane risk-of-bias assessment tool covers some important potential bias domains for clinical trials (i.e., randomisation process, deviation from intended interventions, missing outcome data, measurement of outcomes, and selective reporting) [5].

Standards of Adaptive Trial Designs

Statistical Design

The most important requirement of adaptive trial designs is pre-specification of adaptations and the statistical analysis plan [9–11]. The design should be provided in sufficient detail for

Table 12.1 Minimum standards for adaptive trial designs and master protocols
The minimum standards for adaptive trial designs and master protocols presented in this table are based on the authors' review of the regulatory guidance documents, peer reviewed publications, and experience working in the field of clinical trials.

Standards for adaptive trial designs and master protocols
Pre-specification of adaptations and statistical analysis plan
Control of false error rates
Early stakeholder engagement for buy-in and planning
Plans for infrastructure, operational, and logistical management considerations
Firewall of communication and information flow during the conduct and other measures to prevent operational biases
Transparent reporting of trial findings in accordance with the reporting guidelines
Established mechanisms for trial reporting

the trial to be implemented easily and to allow for a meaningful interpretation of the trial findings for the end users. The specific plans should outline the possible adaptation(s), the timing and frequency of interim analyses, and decision rules [12]. It is possible for the trial to be designed with multiple types of adaptations and decisions, so the details on the interim analyses should include what adaptation(s) should be made as well as when and how each adaptation will be made. The timing and frequency of interim analyses should be specific in terms of the number of patients enrolled, the number of patients evaluated, the number of events, or calendar time.

For each planned adaptation, its corresponding decision rule should be specified with details for the statistical analysis. This should include not only the details for the statistical model itself but also the definition of the analysis population and the endpoint that the decision rules are based on. It is critical that the endpoint is specified instead of the outcome. The term 'outcome' refers to the measured variable (e.g., death), whereas the term 'endpoint' refers to the analysed parameter (mortality status at 90 days) in which the decision rules will be based on. It is possible that an endpoint being used for adaptations may be an intermediate endpoint of the primary endpoint of the trial [13]. In such case, the details on both intermediate and primary endpoints should be pre-specified [13, 14].

The design of adaptive trial designs requires a priori evaluation and characterisation of operating characteristics and statistical properties of adaptations [15]. In adaptive trial designs, potential inflation in type I error rate due to multiple testing (multiplicity) can occur. The expected type I error rate of the trial design with the planned adaptations should be assessed to ensure that the type I error rate can be controlled at the nominal level. The statistical properties of adaptations for classical group sequential designs (e.g., O'Brien–Fleming stopping boundary) can be determined analytically in closed form expressions, so they generally do not require the use of statistical simulations [16]. Clinical trial simulation will be required for other clinical trials with more complex adaptive trial designs.

It is generally recommended to explore the operating characteristics of multiple scenarios with varying treatment effects and event rates [11, 12]. This should include the null hypothesis scenario, where the treatment is assumed to have no treatment effect, to estimate the expected type I error rate. The simulation of multiple null hypothesis scenarios with varying control event rates will be required to demonstrate the control of the false positive error rate [12]. Such demonstration of the type I error rate control is generally mandated for clinical trials, especially those that are being done for registrational purposes [11, 12]. As previously discussed in Chapter 5, we also recommend the clinical trial simulation to explore the effects of enrolment rate, dropout rate, missing data, and other parameters related to the trial progress and quality on its expected performance. This is important since the rate of information and the quality of the data collection will affect the decisions being made for the interim analysis and in turn can have a greater effect on the study performance.

Stakeholder Engagement

While flexibility afforded by adaptive trial designs can greatly add efficiency to the clinical trial, the resulting trial design can be complicated. There is a greater requirement for early stakeholder engagement to ensure that key stakeholders understand the trial design and to address potential issues of concerns during the design stage. Identification of stakeholders for engagement in the design stage is critical. Key stakeholders likely include investigators, research staff, funding agencies, ethics review boards, regulatory agencies, Data Safety and Monitoring Board (DSMB), patient representatives, and members of the scientific community. Communication of the adaptive trial designs should be done with all stakeholders to ensure that there is acceptance of the trial design. Early engagement with the stakeholders can likely improve the overall research efforts, and having the stakeholder buy-in from patient advocates and research staff may even improve the uptake and delivery of the complex trial design. In academic settings, unfortunately based on our personal experience, it is a common practice for the statistician to be engaged after the trial has begun or just a couple of days before the grant proposal is submitted to the granting agency. This should be avoided in all clinical trials, especially when clinical trial simulation is required, since simulation will often require time in advance.

Trial Infrastructure, Logistical, and Operational Considerations

The successful implementation of any clinical trial requires careful planning and considerations for logistical and operational management. For clinical trials using adaptive trial designs, it is likely that more complex trial infrastructure will be required. For any adaptation to be made, we need to ensure that the data on which the adaptation will be based can be collected and processed in a timely, accurate manner. This will increase the demands for timely and accurate data capture and processing to ensure interim analyses can be conducted with high-quality data. For trials using response adaptive randomisation, a centralised randomisation system that can change the allocation probabilities over time will be required.

Adaptive trials should plan how adaptations will be implemented. A successful implementation of clinical trials relies on integrating inputs from multiple personnel who will be responsible for day-to-day procedures and management of the trial. The data management and other trial infrastructure should tested before the trial begins [17]. For instance, if the study allows for early dropping of intervention arms, there should be a plan to address the change in drug supply to support the planned adaptation. If sample size re-estimation is planned, if possible, it may be beneficial not to inform the sponsor and the study team regarding the new enrolment target after the interim. However, this may not be feasible in some settings, especially if additional funding is required to carry out the larger trial.

For all adaptive trial designs, there should be considerations for operational bias with plans for how to limit the communication of the interim results and adaptations that may be made. Considerations of measures to prevent operational bias will require proper oversight through well-thought-out governance model. Interim analyses can reveal some information about the performance of the experimental intervention. Knowledge of such trial adaptations that may have occurred can reveal some information regarding the observed treatment effect. Measures to mitigate such operational biases in adaptive clinical trials will require a strict communication and information flow structure from individuals who will conduct the unblinded analyses and review the unblinded data. There should be a firewall in trial data and information. People with financial conflicts of interest or personal conflicts of interest should be distanced and firewalled from the trial results. The access to the trial data and information should be limited to the members of the independent statistical analysis centre and independent DSMB, who are free from conflict of interest [18].

Reporting Practices

Reporting standard guidelines for conventional randomised clinical trials apply to clinical trials using adaptive trial designs [3, 4, 19]. There is a recently developed extension of the CONSORT statement for adaptive trials [9, 10]. The Adaptive designs CONSORT Extension (ACE) statement outlines several important reporting considerations that have already been mentioned as design and conduct practices. For instance, the type of adaptive trial design used with statistical analysis details should be reported (items 3b and 7b) as well as outcomes used for adaptations (item 6a) and the operating characteristics (item 7a) [9, 10]. The specific reporting guidelines for adaptive trial designs from ACE statement is summarised in Table 12.2.

Table 12.2 A summary of the adaptive designs CONSORT Extension (ACE) statement [9, 10]

Item number	Details
1b	Include the word 'adaptive' in the content or at least as a key word
3b	Provide details of the pre-planned adaptations and statistical details in the Trial Design section of Methods
6a	Indicate outcome measures used to inform adaptations with rationale in the Outcomes section of Methods
7b	Interim analyses and stopping rules in the Sample Size and Operating Characteristics section of Methods
11c	Measures to safeguard and minimise operational biases during the trial in the Blinding section of Randomisation
12a	Statistical methods for adaptations in the Statistical Methods section
12b	Estimation and inference methods in the Statistical Methods section
14b	Explain why the trial was stopped in the Recruitment and Adaptations section of Results
14c	Specify what adaptations were made in the Recruitment and Adaptations section of Results
17c	Report interim results in Outcomes and Estimation section of Results
24b	Provide where standardised operating procedures (SAP) and other trial documents can be accessed

Similar to other reporting guidelines, the ACE was created to help researchers write reports that contain the minimum set of information needed to allow readers to clearly understand what was planned and found in a study. In other words, this is just a reporting guideline and a checklist for the minimum. Reporting guideline checklists are not always indicative of the quality of research [20]. When reporting and evaluating a report or publication reporting the methods and results from an adaptive clinical trial, understanding the context for each clinical question is important. For this, the readers will often be required to think and reason outside the checkboxes. We encourage the readers to do so.

Standards of Master Protocols

Design Practices

The design of master protocols should follow similar standards of methodological rigour as conventional and adaptive clinical trials. For basket, umbrella, and platform trials being conducted with adaptive trial designs, the same standard of pre-specifications of adaptations and demonstration of type I error rate will generally apply. Even though simulation may not be necessary when less complex trial designs are used, we recommend adopting the simulation-guided design planning process [15]. Early stakeholder engagement is critical. As stated before, early engagement with statisticians and other methodologists will be required. Clinical trial simulation is often more complicated and time-consuming than sample size calculations for a fixed sample trial design.

In addition to the statistical considerations, the importance of operational planning will be critically high for clinical trials using master protocols, since these trials tend to be larger and longer term (perpetual in nature), and often involve biomarkers [21, 22]. Building the robust trial infrastructure and networks of sites and partners will be critical for successful and effective management and implementation of complex trial designs. In the setting of platform trials, there will be iterative and overlapping cycles of planning and execution since interventions are able to enter and leave the platform at different times [23–25]. It is likely that many operational partners may have never participated in clinical trials where existing interventions are dropped and new ones are added, so they will require training and education on the practical implications of platform trials. There can be considerable variability in the workflow and workload over time. This will make budgeting difficult. Regardless, the ability to be flexible and nimble in services will be needed to adapt to the dynamic nature of platform trials.

In the setting of biomarker-guided basket, umbrella, or platform trials, there is no shortage of challenges. Recruitment can be difficult, especially when rare biomarker group(s) are being targeted, so high screening failure and low eligibility rates should be anticipated and properly budgeted for [26]. Biospecimen samples collection, processing, and analysis should be properly monitored and documented for good internal audit trails [27]. While having a centralised laboratory can be ideal, this may not always be feasible. The laboratory staff performing these biomarker assays should be trained with Good Clinical Practices and operate under the standardised operating procedures when performing these biomarker assays [27].

Conduct Practices

During the conduct of clinical trials, especially in the case of platform trials, some information about executed adaptations, treatment effects, and other information about the trial (e.g., baseline control event rate, dropout rate) may become known to the public. In the case of non-platform clinical trials, information can be firewalled and better guarded, with the data and interim information being limited to an unblinded independent statistical analysis centre and Data and Safety Monitory Board who will conduct and review the pre-specified interim analyses. This may not always be possible in platform trials given their perpetual nature. For instance, findings on the initially available interventions may become available and reveal information about the control group even when other interventions are being evaluated. While this information is on the non-concurrent control arm, this does reveal information about the trial.

The potential for information leakage needs to be minimised as much as possible [28]. The decision to add new interventions or stop them from being added should not be made based on such information [28]. The decision on what interventions should be made and other aspects of the trial modifications should be made by a group independent of substantial conflict of interest. If a given intervention is found to be effective in a specific biomarker sub-type but is still being evaluated in other groups, the scientific communication of the results should perhaps be delayed until the intervention is no longer active to preserve scientific integrity. Previous platform trials have pre-specified the governance structure to include the central dissemination committee that determines the amount of information that can be publicly shared. This may be required to ensure that the scientific integrity of the ongoing trial can be preserved.

Reporting Practices

The reporting standard guidelines and risk-of-bias assessment tools for conventional and adaptive clinical trials apply to clinical trials using the master protocol framework. As adaptive trial designs are often utilised in basket, umbrella, and platform trials [21, 22], the reporting standards discussed in the section above, particularly the ACE statement, will apply. Since multiple research questions can be evaluated in clinical trials using the master protocol framework, it is usual that there will be multiple publications with each publication reporting the results on the comparison of a single intervention. The assessment of a single publication out of platform trial or other master protocol studies may not differ from other clinical trials. However, platform, basket, and umbrella trials will result in multiple publications, and each trial will contain a considerable body of materials [14, 21, 22]. They likely cannot be fully digested by reading only the abstract or even a single publication. These trials may pose readership burden for the clinical readers, so making sense of these trials can be more challenging. Having a website where all the publications and reports can be centralised will help with the reporting of the clinical trial. Having a trial website also is helpful to ensure that research staff can remain aware of the latest active version of the protocol. Providing visual aids and linking the recorded oral presentations can also be helpful for communication purposes.

Given the perpetual or long-term nature of platform trials, the trial may be more likely to face unavoidable situations that prompt modifications to it (extenuating circumstances) [29]. Examples of extenuating circumstances may include natural disasters, civil unrest, or other externalities that make modifications unavoidable [29]. For example, Randomized, Embedded, Multifactorial Adaptive Platform Trial for Community-Acquired Pneumonia (REMAP-CAP) halted the enrolment to the two hydrocortisone arms being evaluated as part of the corticosteroid therapeutic domains on 17 June 2020 [30]. This came about following the announcement on the mortality benefits of dexamethasone in patients with COVID-19 receiving either invasive mechanical ventilation or supplemental oxygen in the RECOVERY trial [31]. While the pre-specified statistical thresholds in the analysis plan were not met for either of the two hydrocortisone regimens being evaluated, the REMAP-CAP made the decision to halt the intervention groups due to such an external factor, while being unblinded to the data at the time of their decision [30]. The investigators have stated that the unplanned change was unavoidable.

In situations of extenuating circumstances, the investigators and the readers can refer to the CONSORT and the SPIRIT (Standard Protocol Items: Recommendations for Interventional Trials) Extension for RCTs Revised in Extenuating Circumstances (CONSERVE) 2021 statement [29]. This is a framework that can be used for reporting purposes and also for evaluation of the effect of modifications that the trial investigators have made [29]. The CONSERVE 2021 statement outlines communication of extenuating circumstances, parties responsible for planning, reviewing, and approving the trial modifications, and modifications to the trial or the environment as part of the mitigation strategies for the extenuating circumstance [29].

Conclusion

When designed and executed with methodological rigour, clinical trials using adaptive trial designs or a master protocol framework have the potential to address many of the limitations associated with conventional clinical trials (e.g., two-arm trials). These clinical trials often must be undertaken carefully to prevent statistical and operational bias and be reported with adequate transparency to improve the interpretability of their findings. In this chapter, we have discussed standards for the design, conduct, and reporting of adaptive trial designs and master protocols. Our discussion in this chapter has included several standard reporting guidelines and risk-of-bias assessment tools, but we encourage readers to review articles on adaptive trial designs and master protocols with an open mind. Undoubtedly, these guidelines and tools are important checklists, but understanding the context of each clinical question will be critical.

References

1. Friedman LM, Furberg C, DeMets DL, Reboussin D, Granger CB. *Fundamentals of Clinical Trials*. Springer; 2015.

2. Chan AW, Tetzlaff JM, Altman DG, et al. SPIRIT 2013 statement: defining standard protocol items for clinical trials. *Ann Intern Med*. 2013;**158**(3):200–207.

3. Schulz KF, Altman DG, Moher D, Group C. CONSORT 2010 statement: updated guidelines for reporting parallel group randomised trials. *Trials*. 2010;**11**:32.

4. Schulz KF, Altman DG, Moher D, Group C. CONSORT 2010 statement: updated guidelines for reporting parallel group randomised trials. *BMJ*. 2010;**340**:c332.

5. Sterne JAC, Savovic J, Page MJ, et al. RoB 2: a revised tool for assessing risk of bias in randomised trials. *BMJ*. 2019;**366**:l4898.

6. Park JJH, Dron L, Mills EJ. Moving forward in clinical research with master protocols. *Contemp Clin Trials*. 2021;**106**:106438.

7. Bhatt DL, Mehta C. Adaptive designs for clinical trials. *N Engl J Med*. 2016;**375** (1):65–74.

8. Van Norman GA. Phase II trials in drug development and adaptive trial design. *JACC Basic Transl Sci*. 2019;4(3):428–37.

9. Dimairo M, Pallmann P, Wason J, et al. The adaptive designs CONSORT extension

(ACE) statement: a checklist with explanation and elaboration guideline for reporting randomised trials that use an adaptive design. *Trials*. 2020; **21**(1):528.

10. Dimairo M, Pallmann P, Wason J, et al. The Adaptive designs CONSORT Extension (ACE) statement: a checklist with explanation and elaboration guideline for reporting randomised trials that use an adaptive design. *BMJ*. 2020;**369**:m115.

11. Detry MA, Lewis RJ, Broglio KR, et al. Standards for the design, conduct, and evaluation of adaptive randomized clinical trials. Patient-Centered Outcomes Research Institute (PCORI), 2012.

12. United States Department of Health and Human Services, Food and Drug Administration. *Adaptive Designs for Clinical Trials of Drugs and Biologics. Guidance for Industry*. Center for Biologics Evaluation and Research (CBER). 2019.

13. Sydes MR, Parmar MK, James ND, et al. Issues in applying multi-arm multi-stage methodology to a clinical trial in prostate cancer: the MRC STAMPEDE trial. *Trials*. 2009;**10**:39.

14. Park JJH, Harari O, Dron L, et al. An overview of platform trials with a checklist for clinical readers. *J Clin Epidemiol*. 2020;**125**:1–8.

15. Mayer C, Perevozskaya I, Leonov S, et al. Simulation practices for adaptive trial designs in drug and device development. *Statistics in Biopharmaceutical Research*. 2019;**11**(4):325–35.

16. Thorlund K, Haggstrom J, Park JJ, Mills EJ. Key design considerations for adaptive clinical trials: a primer for clinicians. *BMJ*. 2018;**360**:k698.

17. He W, Kuznetsova OM, Harmer M, et al. Practical considerations and strategies for executing adaptive clinical trials. *DIJ*. 2012;**46**(2):160–74.

18. Fisher MR, Roecker EB, DeMets DL. The role of an independent statistical analysis center in the institutes of health model. *DIJ*. 2001;**35**(1):115–29.

19. Juszczak E, Altman DG, Hopewell S, Schulz K. Reporting of multi-arm

parallel-group randomized trials: extension of the CONSORT 2010 statement. *JAMA*. 2019;**321**(16):1610–20.

20. Logullo P, MacCarthy A, Kirtley S, Collins GS. Reporting guideline checklists are not quality evaluation forms: they are guidance for writing. *Health Sci Rep*. 2020;**3**(2).

21. Park JJH, Siden E, Zoratti MJ, et al. Systematic review of basket trials, umbrella trials, and platform trials: a landscape analysis of master protocols. *Trials*. 2019; **20**(1):572.

22. Siden EG, Park JJ, Zoratti MJ, et al. Reporting of master protocols towards a standardized approach: a systematic review. *Contemp Clin Trials Commun*. 2019;**15**:100406.

23. Schiavone F, Bathia R, Letchemanan K, et al. This is a platform alteration: a trial management perspective on the operational aspects of adaptive and platform and umbrella protocols. *Trials*. 2019; **20**(1):264.

24. Morrell L, Hordern J, Brown L, et al. Mind the gap? The platform trial as a working environment. *Trials*. 2019; **20**(1):1–6.

25. Hague D, Townsend S, Masters L, et al. Changing platforms without stopping the train: experiences of data management and data management systems when adapting platform protocols by adding and closing comparisons. *Trials*. 2019; **20**(1):1–16.

26. Park JJH, Hsu G, Siden EG, Thorlund K, Mills EJ. An overview of precision oncology basket and umbrella trials for clinicians. *CA Cancer J Clin*. 2020;**70** (2):125–37.

27. Antoniou M, Kolamunnage-Dona R, Wason J, et al. Biomarker-guided trials: challenges in practice. *Contemp Clin Trials Commun*. 2019;**16**:100493.

28. Park JJH, Detry MA, Murthy S, Guyatt G, Mills EJ. How to use and interpret the results of a platform trial: users' guide to the medical literature. *JAMA*. 2022;**327** (1):67–74.

29. Orkin AM, Gill PJ, Ghersi D, et al. Guidelines for reporting trial protocols and

completed trials modified due to the COVID-19 pandemic and other extenuating circumstances: the CONSERVE 2021 statement. *JAMA*. 2021;**326**(3):257–65.

30. Angus DC, Derde L, Al-Beidh F, et al. Effect of hydrocortisone on mortality and organ support in patients with severe COVID-19: The REMAP-CAP COVID-19 corticosteroid domain randomized clinical trial. *JAMA*. 2020;**324**(13):1317–29.

31. Recovery Collaborative Group, Horby P, Lim WS, Emberson JR, et al. Dexamethasone in hospitalized patients with Covid-19. *N Engl J Med*. 2021;**384**(8):693–704.

Common Misconceptions of Adaptive Trial Designs and Master Protocols

Chapter

13

Jay J. H. Park, Edward J. Mills, and J. Kyle Wathen

Key Points of This Chapter

In this chapter, we review 10 common misconceptions of adaptive trial designs and master protocols encountered during our collective experience in teaching and working in the field of clinical trial research.

The key points of this chapter are:

- There is no such thing as a free lunch. There will be trade-offs between every design choice that is made for the clinical investigation.
- There are situations in which clinical trials with adaptive trial designs and master protocols will be highly beneficial. There will also be situations in which they will not.
- The foremost step to good clinical trial research is to ask important research questions and answer them reliably. Adaptive trial designs and master protocol frameworks are merely tools for clinical investigation. These methodological tools should be forced to shape and fit the research question.

Introduction

During our collective experience in teaching, designing, and helping to conduct clinical trials with adaptive trial designs and master protocol frameworks, we have frequently encountered the 10 misconceptions that are outlined in Table 13.1. This chapter reviews the misconceptions to clarify them for readers.

Table 13.1 Common misconceptions of adaptive trial designs and master protocols

Misconceptions	Facts
1. Clinical trials that stop early are problematic.	Sequential designs are statistically valid and can provide statistical, practical, and ethical advantages to clinical trial research.
2. Adaptive trial designs have a high risk of bias.	Adaptive trial designs are heavily protocol driven. They are not an excuse for making post hoc unplanned changes.
3. Being adaptive and Bayesian is synonymous.	The difference between Bayesian and frequentist statistics stems from their different interpretation of probability. There are advantages to Bayesian statistics, but frequentist statistics can be used to guide adaptive clinical trials and master protocols.

Table 13.1 (cont.)

Misconceptions	Facts
4. There are benefits to response adaptive randomisation	For right questions, response adaptive randomisation can have important benefits, but if poorly planned and executed, they lead to undesirable and even detrimental effects on the trial's performance.
5. Adaptive trial designs are better than conventional trials.	There is no such thing as a free lunch, and no design is without its limitations. No design, adaptive or not, should be used as a default choice.
6. Master protocols are studies.	Master protocols are merely protocol documents that outline plans for basket, umbrella, or platform trials.
7. 'Master protocol' studies are randomised clinical trials.	Not all clinical trials using the master protocol framework involve randomisation.
8. Adaptive trial designs and master protocols are synonymous.	Not all clinical trials using a master protocol framework use adaptive trial designs. There are examples of fixed and adaptive basket, umbrella, and platform trials.
9. Platform trials use response adaptive randomisation.	Platform trials refer to clinical trials that are designed to add new interventions into an ongoing clinical trial. Response adaptive randomisation is not a defining feature of platform trials.
10. Platform trials are Bayesian.	There are examples of both high-quality frequentist and Bayesian platform trials. Platform trials do not need to be limited to Bayesian statistics.

Misconceptions of Adaptive Trial Designs

Misconception 1: Clinical Trials That Stop Early Are Problematic

There have been several influential articles that have argued against sequential designs [1–4]. In these articles, early stopping rules are described as problematic and even dangerous to participants, clinicians, and society [1–4]. Their recommendations even included that independent Data Safety and Monitoring Boards (DSMB) should not review unblinded efficacy data but rather focus on monitoring harm [3]. This school of thought is central to the fact that trials that stop early for an apparent benefit, on average, will result in biased treatment estimates [1–4]. It is true that the point estimates will be biased and can be higher than the true effect in such situations [5, 6]. Since a smaller dataset is available at the time of interim analysis, the estimation will be less precise. The opposition to sequential designs has argued that this is problematic because the primary purpose of clinical trials should be to obtain an accurate estimate of the benefits for a given experimental therapy [1]. An accurate estimation of treatment effect is desirable, but in reality, this is often undesirable and impractical.

Clinical trials are not designed with the goal of estimation. Instead, clinical trial design follows a hypothesis–test framework, in which the primary goal is to determine whether a given therapy is comparatively more efficacious than one or more other groups while controlling for false error rates [7]. We control for potential inflation of the false positive error rate (multiplicity) by using a stringent statistical threshold for early stopping; therefore, even at the expense of biased point estimation, such sequential designs remain valid. It is also the case that small clinical trials are prone to overestimating the treatment effect, regardless of whether the trial had stopped early or recruited to its final target sample size [8]. A conventional trial will have a biased estimate when compared against a trial that is larger [8].

There are often financial and other feasibility constraints that limit the size of the trial. To optimise the treatment effect estimation, it is likely that an incredibly large sample size will be required. Also, it could not be feasible to recruit enough patients with such magnitude, and this could even reduce the resources that could be used for other research questions. As we have seen during the COVID-19 pandemic with vaccine development, getting to a statistically conclusive finding more quickly is beneficial to society at large, even at the expense of larger uncertainty in the estimated treatment effects. Given finite resources, funding one trial means there will be less funding for another trial or other research questions, leading to a smaller number of experimental therapies being evaluated [9].

Stopping a trial early does raise important administrative challenges. Once a trial has been stopped at the recommendation of the DSMB, usually based on a finding relevant to the a priori chosen primary outcome, the local or national ethics committee must be made aware of it. If, after stopping the trial, the investigators or DSMB feels the trial should be restarted, this will require a discussion or possibly reapplication with the ethics committee. Such stoppages are unlikely to result in restarting the trial.

There should be no one-size-fits-all approach to clinical research. There are instances in which early stopping is appropriate. Early stopping can provide ethical advantages for patients inside or outside the trial by reaching the conclusion earlier, leading to benefits, such as fewer patients randomised to the inferior study arm and resource savings that could be diverted to other research questions [8]. An aim to answer the research questions with minimal resources and time is appropriate and pragmatic.

Misconception 2: Adaptive Trial Designs Have a High Risk of Bias

Among researchers and funders, there are often negative attitudes and conservatism towards adaptive trial designs and insistence on conventional fixed sample designs [10, 11]. There are concerns regarding the robustness of adaptive trial designs, but many of these concerns may stem from the fact that researchers and funders are often unfamiliar with adaptive trial designs [10, 12]. Adaptive trial designs can certainly be more complex and require a team of investigators with methodological and statistical expertise and experience [13]. Communication of adaptive trial designs can be difficult, since many lack the knowledge and experience, and more education and training opportunities are needed [10]. Incomprehension should not be confused with perceived bias. Complex trials often are planned and executed with methodological rigour closely following many of the standards of adaptive trial designs [14–16].

Contrary to some common beliefs, adaptive trial designs are not an excuse for post hoc unplanned changes to the trial. Adaptive trial designs are and should be protocol driven. The flexibility afforded by adaptive trial designs is planned during the design stage, with the detailed plans and justification being outlined in the protocol, statistical analysis plan, and adaptive trial design report (or simulation report) [17–19]. When post hoc unplanned changes are made, clinical trials are prone to biases, regardless of whether adaptive trial designs are used or not, especially when these changes are made based on unblinded data. Of course, there can be extenuating circumstances that make unplanned changes unavoidable, especially when trials are conducted over a long period of time. By coming up with formalised plans for how the design will respond and adapt to the accumulating information, adaptive trial designs can minimise the need for post hoc changes in comparison to the conventional designs [18].

Misconception 3: Being Adaptive and Bayesian Is Synonymous

Advocates of Bayesian statistics, 'Bayesians', have long argued that Bayesian philosophy is ideally suited to adapt to accumulating information during clinical trials with adaptive trial designs [20]. The use of the Bayes theorem allows us to formally incorporate prior information regarding treatment effects, and when new information (e.g., data) is presented, our beliefs can be updated accordingly [20, 21]. Bayesians often argue that this is how humans naturally think, but psychologists in the past have argued that this is not always the case [22]. Our confirmation biases can lead to deviations from such Bayesian updates [23].

The distinction between Bayesians and frequentists is not always clear, but they both share the common goal of learning from data about the world around us with different interpretations of probability [24]. The p-value and the frequentist philosophy have been increasingly criticised for their misuse, leading to some journals recently banning its use [25, 26]. We have seen increasing numbers of post hoc re-analysis of clinical trials with Bayesian analyses that all end with a common conclusion that being Bayesian is better [27]. Certainly, the outputs of Bayesian analyses, such as credible intervals and posterior probability of superiority, can offer much more straightforward interpretation than their frequentist counterparts in confidence intervals and p-values [28]. Frequentist statistical infrequence requires adjustment on the basis of their intended trial design [29]. Whereas with the Bayesian approach, no adjustment to the posterior is needed, regardless of when the analysis is carried out [30]. The posterior distribution is oblivious to multiple analyses and stopping rules, and because of that, Bayesian decision rules, in principle, do not need to be adjusted [20, 30]. Of course, this does not mean being Bayesian could be used as an excuse for poor planning and execution.

We often call adaptive trial designs with decision rules that are defined in terms of posterior and predictive probabilities 'Bayesian clinical trials'. In practice, as regulations currently stand, clinical trialists determine these decision rules to meet the type I error rate requirement by simulating under the null effect scenario that assumes that there is no treatment effect (e.g., RR = 1.00) [17]. Regulatory agencies, such as the U.S. Food and Drug Administration, will require all registrational trials to control for type I error rate at a nominal level (e.g., 2.5% one-sided) [31–33]. In accordance with their pre-specified interim analyses plan, Bayesian decision rules (e.g., superiority and futility thresholds) are calibrated using simulations to meet type I error rate requirements, while trying to optimise statistical power (type II error) in reasonable sample sizes that can be recruited. Right or wrong, Bayesian and frequentist clinical trials are often required to meet the same frequentist error constraints.

Misconception 4: There Are Benefits to Response Adaptive Randomisation

Among statisticians, response adaptive randomisation is certainly not without controversy [34]. In our experience, many clinical investigators will ask for response adaptive randomisation due to its ethical appeal. Response adaptive randomisation can theoretically make randomisation more comfortable by adapting the allocation ratio to the treatment arms that are performing better [35]. Even when they are unproven, there is often preference towards experimental therapies, so the use of response adaptive randomisation can be appealing [36]. Response adaptive randomisation has the potential to reduce the size of the control group that often is perceived to be inferior at the design and recruitment stage, despite the experimental nature of clinical trials.

Response adaptive randomisation can lead to unwanted results. For instance, in two-arm settings, response adaptive randomisation has been shown to create sample size imbalance between the treatment and control groups in the wrong direction, in which more patients end up being randomised to the inferior group [37]. Imbalance in sample size can result in lower statistical power and less reliable statistical inference than a randomised clinical trial with equal allocation [37]. The use of response adaptive randomisation in multi-arm trial settings can have better performance, given that allocation to the control arm is adequately maintained or even increased throughout the trial [38]. Since the allocation to the control is often required, this may not reduce the number of patients who end up being randomised to the control.

Response adaptive randomisation also can pose operational challenges and will require more complex clinical trial infrastructure [39]. Commonly used web-based randomisation systems, such as REDCap, only support fixed randomisation. More complex and costly solutions will likely be required to carry out response adaptive randomisation design. It cannot be emphasised enough that there is no such thing as a free lunch. The pros and cons of each design choice including response adaptive randomisation should be carefully weighed during the design stage. There will be situations in which response adaptive randomisation will be highly beneficial, and there will be other situations in which it will not be.

Misconception 5: Adaptive Trials Are Better Than Conventional Trials

Perception of adaptive trial designs is often divided into two camps: strong sceptics and strong proponents. While we remain enthusiasts of adaptive trial designs, it is important to point out that adaptive trial designs are not always useful [40]. Adaptive trial designs require reliable information to be available at an interim, and they often use a single endpoint to guide the decision for adaptations. Optimising the trial design based on a single endpoint may even harm secondary analyses on secondary endpoints and sub-group analyses [41]. Even if the type I error rate can be strictly controlled for, there may be no way to avoid the fact that there will be less information that will be provided [41]. Flexibility and resource savings afforded by adaptive trial designs will result in reduced data on secondary efficacy endpoints and safety data that are critical for risk-benefit assessment of a given experimental therapy [41].

Decisions for adaptations are made on interim data from the enrolled participants. They must have been followed up for enough time for the endpoint that is being used to guide the decision for adaptations to be observed. When adaptations are made, the changes in the trial design affect the future participants, not the participants who have already been enrolled. For instance, a two-arm trial with sequential design can end early, but the patients, who have already been randomised, will usually finish their planned clinical follow-up. When allocation

Table 13.2 Comparison of recruitment and follow-up time

Time (month)	Recruitment: 50 patients/month & 2 months' follow-up		Recruitment: 100 patients/month & 2 months' follow-up	
	No. of patients enrolled	No. of outcomes observed	No. of patients enrolled	No. of outcomes observed
0	0	0	0	0
1	50	0	100	0
2	100	0	200	0
3	150	50	300	100
4	200	100	400	200
5	250	150	**500**	**300**
6	300	200		400
7	350	250		500
8	**400**	**300**		
9	450	350	Recruitment reached	
10	500	400		Follow-up completed
11		450		
12	Recruitment reached	500		
13		Trial follow-up		

Note: This is the same two-arm trial with an enrolment target of 500 patients who will each be followed up for 2 months. A single interim analysis is planned after 300 patients have finished their follow-up.

ratios are altered in response adaptive randomisation, this affects how the incoming participants will be randomised. Patients who have already been randomised will not be re-randomised.

It might not always feasible to carry out adaptations. This is the case if the primary endpoint of interest takes a long time to measure, especially when there is comparatively fast recruitment [40]. Let us consider an example of a two-arm trial with two varying recruitment rates of 50 patients per month versus 100 patients per month, as outlined in Table 13.2. This hypothetical trial is designed to recruit up to 500 patients, who will each be followed up for 2 months. There is a single interim analysis planned after 300th patient has finished their follow-up.

With the slower recruitment rate of 50 patients per month, the 300th patient will finish their follow-up around month 8. Since 400 patients have already been enrolled, there will be a potential savings of 100 patients with early stopping. With the faster recruitment (100 patients per month), the 300th patient will finish their follow-up around month 5. Since the maximum recruitment target has already been reached, it will be feasible to carry out the planned interim analysis. There would be no savings in such a case. This is a very simplified example, but it should illustrate how most adaptive trial designs will require the endpoint for adaptations to be observed sufficiently quickly in comparison to the recruitment [40].

The example above highlights how the magnitude of benefits with planned adaptations depends on the interim analyses plan. If the interim analysis is planned earlier than the 300th observed patient, the feasibility and magnitude of sample size savings can both be increased. The magnitude of potential efficiency usually does become greater with more aggressive interim analyses plans (e.g., smaller burn-in and multiple interims). However, it should be noted that an aggressive interim analysis plan does not always lead to greater savings [18, 40].

It is possible to design adaptive trials to use an endpoint that is quick to measure for interim analyses. If an intermediate endpoint being used for interim analyses is different from the primary endpoint of interest, this improves the feasibility of the trial. This requires that the information on the intermediate endpoint must be useful in predicting what would occur if the trial were to continue to the end. As key assumptions, two endpoints should be correlated, and measurable improvement in the intermediate endpoint should lead to a measurable improvement in the primary endpoint, and vice versa [42].

Operational burden in terms of both administrative and logistical complexity is often overlooked [16, 43]. To carry out an interim analysis, the interim data must be processed and analysed relatively quickly under high standards. Albeit manageable, conducting an adaptive clinical trial with even a single interim analysis will be more difficult than conducting a conventional clinical trial, where there is only one final analysis at the end. In addition to statistical complexities, the trial design with more aggressive interim analyses plans will raise its operational complexity and be more difficult to manage and implement properly. Implementation challenges are not always easy for the research staff to manage [44].

Although adaptive trial designs have received substantial attention in recent years, they are not without limitations. The discussion for this misconception is not to deter the use of adaptive trial designs. However, it is important to realise that there is no such thing as a free lunch. We encourage the investigators to weigh the pros and cons when conducting a clinical trial. Adaptive trial designs are merely a tool to help answer the research question of interest. These tools should not be forced into the research question. Rather, the research questions should guide the decision on what specific design to use. The criteria to good clinical research are foremost to ask important questions and to answer them reliably [45]. No design, whether adaptive or not, should be used as a default choice. Every research question deserves a thorough investigation and consideration of the pros and cons when selecting the most optimal design choice for a given question.

Misconceptions of Master Protocols

Misconception 6: Master Protocols Are Studies

The misused terminology of master protocols is common [46]. The terminology of 'master protocols' refers to a series of protocol documents developed to coordinate efforts in evaluation of one or more therapies [31, 47, 48]. The master protocol is used to standardise and harmonise clinical trial evaluations across multiple interventions that end up being evaluated within the common overall trial structure. Master protocols are often mistakenly referred to as clinical trials [46]. Clinical trials that use the master protocol framework, such as basket trials, umbrella trials, and platform trials, are the trials themselves. Master protocols simply refer to protocol documents developed to conduct these clinical trials.

Misconception 7: 'Master Protocol' Studies Are Randomised Clinical Trials

Basket trials, umbrella trials, and platform trials are intervention studies in which human volunteers receive specific interventions and follow prospectively over time according to the plans outlined in their master protocol. The use of randomisation is common in umbrella trials and platform trials, but it is not a methodological requirement that defines these clinical trials [48]. It is possible for basket, umbrella, and platform trials to be conducted as non-randomised and randomised clinical trials [46, 48, 49]. In fact, most basket trials that have been conducted thus far are done so as exploratory phase I or IIA trials using single-arm (non-randomised) designs [48]. Basket trials are most frequently conducted in oncology and uses the Simon two-stage design to identify a targeted therapy with a promising tumour response rate. With increasing emphasis on precision oncology, there have been examples of tumour- and histology-agnostic therapies that have received regulatory approval based on non-randomised basket trial evidence [49]. However, since it is quite difficult to recruit enough patients with the targeted biomarkers, basket trials often do not use randomisation [46, 48].

Misconception 8: Adaptive Trial Designs and Master Protocols Are Synonymous

The use of adaptive trial designs is common in basket trials, umbrella trials, and platform trials. In basket trials, the Simon two-stage design uses the results of the interim results at the first stage to determine whether continuation into the second stage is warranted [50]. Sequential designs and response adaptive randomisation are two common types of adaptive trial designs that are used in adaptive platform trials [42, 51]. However, the use of these adaptive trial designs is not a defining feature for basket, umbrella, and platform trials [46]. We know that adaptive trial designs have been used in 'non-master protocol' clinical trials for several decades [19, 52]. There have also been examples of non-adaptive basket, umbrella, and platform trials [48].

The term, 'adaptive trial designs' refers to a group of different designs that have outlined pre-specified plans for how the trial will respond to the accumulating data [19, 52]. This does not meet the defining features of basket, umbrella, and platform trials. The defining feature of basket trials is the evaluation of one or more therapies that aim to target specific molecular alterations and/or other predictive risk factors (treatable traits) [47, 49, 53]. The defining feature of umbrella trials is evaluation of multiple targeted interventions in a single disease that is stratified into multiple sub-studies based on different molecular or predictive risk factors [31, 47–49]. Lastly, platform trials refer to clinical trials that are designed with the flexibility to allow new interventions into an existing trial infrastructure [42, 48, 51].

Misconceptions 9 & 10: Platform Trials Use Response Adaptive Randomisation and Platform Trials Are Bayesian

There are many examples of non-platform clinical trials and adaptive platform trials that are designed with response adaptive randomisation [54, 55]. Response adaptive randomisation is simply a method that allows for dynamic allocation ratio [37, 38, 56]. This is not a defining feature of platform trials. Platform trials are clinical trials that allow new interventions to be added [42, 48]. Bayesian statistics have been used in both non-platform and platform trials [19, 42, 48, 52]. It can certainly make communication of the trial results easier, but there is nothing magical about being Bayesian, as discussed in the section above for Misconception 3. There are examples of frequentist and Bayesian platform trials that are high quality [42, 48].

Conclusion

There are common misconceptions that stem across adaptive trial designs and master protocols. Adaptive trial designs are often challenged with affinity towards conventional trial designs. Master protocols are challenged by the lack of standardisation in their terminologies that have attributed to their inconsistent use. For the right research questions and area of clinical research, adaptive trial designs and master protocols can offer several advantages over conventional approaches for clinical trial research. However, this is not always the case. We believe the most important requirement to good quality clinical research is to ask important research questions. Then we can determine what the most optimal design choice will be.

References

1. Mueller PS, Montori VM, Bassler D, Koenig BA, Guyatt GH. Ethical issues in stopping randomized trials early because of apparent benefit. *Ann Int Med.* 2007;**146**(12):878–81.

2. Guyatt GH, Briel M, Glasziou P, Bassler D, Montori VM. Problems of stopping trials early. *BMJ.* 2012;**344**:e3863.

3. Bassler D, Montori VM, Briel M, Glasziou P, Guyatt G. Early stopping of randomized clinical trials for overt efficacy is problematic. *J Clin Epidemiol.* 2008;**61**(3):241–6.

4. Briel M, Bassler D, Wang AT, Guyatt GH, Montori VM. The dangers of stopping a trial too early. *J Bone Joint Surg Am.* 2012;**94**(Suppl 1):56–60.

5. Pocock SJ, Hughes MD. Practical problems in interim analyses, with particular regard to estimation. *Control Clin Trials.* 1989;**10**(4 Suppl):209S–21S.

6. Fan XF, DeMets DL, Lan KK. Conditional bias of point estimates following a group sequential test. *J Biopharm Stat.* 2004;**14**(2):505–30.

7. Goodman SN. Stopping at nothing? Some dilemmas of data monitoring in clinical trials. *Ann Int Med.* 2007;**146**(12):882–7.

8. Viele K, McGlothlin A, Broglio K. Interpretation of clinical trials that stopped early. *Jama.* 2016;**315**(15):1646–7.

9. Flight L, Julious S, Brennan A, Todd S. Expected value of sample information to guide the design of group sequential clinical trials. *Med Decis Making.* 2022;**42**(4):461–73.

10. Dimairo M, Boote J, Julious SA, Nicholl JP, Todd S. Missing steps in a staircase: a qualitative study of the perspectives of key stakeholders on the use of adaptive designs in confirmatory trials. *Trials.* 2015;**16**(1):1–16.

11. Jaki T. Uptake of novel statistical methods for early-phase clinical studies in the UK public sector. *Clin Trials.* 2013;**10**(2):344–6.

12. Madani Kia T, Marshall JC, Murthy S. Stakeholder perspectives on adaptive clinical trials: a scoping review. *Trials.* 2020;**21**(1):539.

13. He W, Kuznetsova OM, Harmer M, et al. Practical considerations and strategies for executing adaptive clinical trials. *DIJ.* 2012;**46**(2):160–74.

14. Dimairo M, Pallmann P, Wason J, et al. The adaptive designs CONSORT extension (ACE) statement: a checklist with explanation and elaboration guideline for reporting randomised trials that use an adaptive design. *Trials.* 2020;**21**(1):528.

15. Dimairo M, Pallmann P, Wason J, et al. The Adaptive designs CONSORT Extension (ACE) statement: a checklist with explanation and elaboration guideline for reporting randomised trials that use an adaptive design. *BMJ.* 2020;**369**:m115.

16. Detry MA, Lewis RJ, Broglio KR, et al. Standards for the design, conduct, and evaluation of adaptive randomized clinical trials. Patient-Centered Outcomes Research Institute (PCORI); 2012.

17. Mayer C, Perevozskaya I, Leonov S, et al. Simulation practices for adaptive trial designs in drug and device development. *Stat Biopharm Res.* 2019;**11**(4):325–35.

18. Thorlund K, Haggstrom J, Park JJ, Mills EJ. Key design considerations for adaptive clinical trials: a primer for clinicians. *BMJ.* 2018;**360**:k698.

19. Bhatt DL, Mehta C. Adaptive designs for clinical trials. *N Engl J Med.* 2016;**375**(1):65–74.

20. Berry DA. Bayesian clinical trials. *Nat Rev Drug Discov.* 2006;**5**(1):27–36.

21. Senn S. You may believe you are a Bayesian but you are probably wrong. Error Statistics Philosophy; 2011.

22. Tversky A, Kahneman D. Judgment under uncertainty: heuristics and biases. *Science.* 1974;**185**(4157):1124–31.

23. Dave C, Wolfe KW. On confirmation bias and deviations from Bayesian updating. Working Paper, University of Pittsburgh; 2004.

24. Johnson AA, Ott MQ, Dogucu M. *Bayes Rules!: An Introduction to Applied Bayesian Modeling.* CRC Press; 2022.

25. Woolston C. Psychology journal bans *P* values. *Nature.* 2015;**519**(7541):9.

26. Singh Chawla D. 'One-size-fits-all' threshold for P values under fire. *Nature News.* 2017.

27. Yarnell CJ, Abrams D, Baldwin MR, et al. Clinical trials in critical care: can a Bayesian approach enhance clinical and scientific decision making? *Lancet Resp Med.* 2021;**9**(2):207–16.

28. Greenland S, Senn SJ, Rothman KJ, et al. Statistical tests, *P* values, confidence intervals, and power: a guide to misinterpretations. *Eur J Epidemiol.* 2016;**31**(4):337–50.

29. Wagenmakers EJ. A practical solution to the pervasive problems of *p* values. *Psychon Bull Rev.* 2007;**14**(5):779–804.

30. Berry DA. Interim analysis in clinical trials: the role of the likelihood principle. *Am Stat.* 1987;**41**(2):117–22.

31. United States Department of Health and Human Services, Food and Drug Administration. *Master Protocols: Efficient Clinical Trial Design Strategies to Expedite Development of Oncology Drugs and Biologics Guidance for Industry.*United States Department of Health and Human Services; 2022. www.fda.gov/media/120721/download.

32. United States Department of Health and Human Services, Food and Drug Administration. *Adaptive Designs for Clinical Trials of Drugs and Biologics. Guidance for Industry.* Center for Biologics Evaluation and Research (CBER). 2019.

33. United States Department of Health and Human Services, Food and Drug Administration. *Master Protocols: Efficient Clinical Trial Design Strategies to Expedite Development of Oncology Drugs and Biologics Guidance for Industry (Draft Guidance).* United States Department of Health and Human Services; 2018 www.fda.gov/downloads/Drugs/GuidanceComplianceRegulatoryInformation/Guidances/UCM621817.pdf

34. Proschan M, Evans S. Resist the temptation of response-adaptive randomization. *Clin Infect Dis.* 2020;**71**(11):3002–4.

35. Angus DC. Optimizing the trade-off between learning and doing in a pandemic. *JAMA.* 2020;**323**(19):1895–6.

36. Meurer WJ, Lewis RJ, Berry DA. Adaptive clinical trials: a partial remedy for the therapeutic misconception? *JAMA.* 2012;**307**(22):2377–8.

37. Thall P, Fox P, Wathen J. Statistical controversies in clinical research: scientific and ethical problems with adaptive randomization in comparative clinical trials. *Ann Oncol.* 2015;**26**(8):1621–8.

38. Viele K, Broglio K, McGlothlin A, Saville BR. Comparison of methods for control allocation in multiple arm studies using response adaptive randomization. *Clin Trials.* 2020;**17**(1):52–60.

39. Zhao W, Durkalski V. Managing competing demands in the implementation of response-adaptive randomization in

a large multicenter phase III acute stroke trial. *Stat Med.* 2014;**33**(23):4043–52.

40. Wason JM, Brocklehurst P, Yap C. When to keep it simple – adaptive designs are not always useful. *BMC Med.* 2019;**17**(1):1–7.

41. Senn S. Being efficient about efficacy estimation. *Stat Biopharm Res.* 2013;**5**(3):204–10.

42. Park JJH, Harari O, Dron L, et al. An overview of platform trials with a checklist for clinical readers. *J Clin Epidemiol.* 2020;**125**:1–8.

43. Hague D, Townsend S, Masters L, et al. Changing platforms without stopping the train: experiences of data management and data management systems when adapting platform protocols by adding and closing comparisons. *Trials.* 2019;**20**(1):1–16.

44. Schiavone F, Bathia R, Letchemanan K, et al. This is a platform alteration: a trial management perspective on the operational aspects of adaptive and platform and umbrella protocols. *Trials.* 2019;**20**(1):264.

45. Yusuf S, Collins R, Peto R. Why do we need some large, simple randomized trials? *Stat Med.* 1984;**3**(4):409–20.

46. Siden EG, Park JJ, Zoratti MJ, et al. Reporting of master protocols towards a standardized approach: a systematic review. *Contemp Clin Trials Commun.* 2019;**15**:100406.

47. Woodcock J, LaVange LM. Master protocols to study multiple therapies, multiple diseases, or both. *N Engl J Med.* 2017;**377**(1):62–70.

48. Park JJH, Siden E, Zoratti MJ, et al. Systematic review of basket trials, umbrella trials, and platform trials: a landscape analysis of master protocols. *Trials.* 2019;**20**(1):572.

49. Park JJH, Hsu G, Siden EG, Thorlund K, Mills EJ. An overview of precision oncology basket and umbrella trials for clinicians. *CA Cancer J Clin.* 2020;**70**(2):125–37.

50. Simon R. Optimal two-stage designs for phase II clinical trials. *Control Clin Trials.* 1989;**10**(1):1–10.

51. Park JJH, Detry MA, Murthy S, Guyatt G, Mills EJ. How to use and interpret the results of a platform trial: users' guide to the medical literature. *JAMA.* 2022;**327**(1):67–74.

52. Bauer P, Bretz F, Dragalin V, Konig F, Wassmer G. Twenty-five years of confirmatory adaptive designs: opportunities and pitfalls. *Stat Med.* 2016;**35**(3):325–47.

53. Bogin V. Master protocols: new directions in drug discovery. *Contemp Clin Trials Commun.* 2020;**18**:100568.

54. Grieve AP. Response-adaptive clinical trials: case studies in the medical literature. *Pharm Stat.* 2017;**16**(1):64–86.

55. Angus DC, Alexander BM, Berry S, et al. Adaptive platform trials: definition, design, conduct and reporting considerations. *Nat Rev Drug Discov.* 2019;**18**(10):797–808.

56. Wathen JK, Thall PF. A simulation study of outcome adaptive randomization in multi-arm clinical trials. *Clin Trials.* 2017;**14**(5):432–40.

Practical Considerations for Adaptive Trial Designs and Master Protocols

Jay J. H. Park, Edward J. Mills, and J. Kyle Wathen

Key Points of This Chapter

In this chapter, we discuss practical considerations of adaptive trial designs and master protocols. The key points of this chapter are:

- Planning adaptive trial designs and master protocols require resources and time. It is best to plan ahead with key stakeholders concerning statistical, content, and operational expertise to make the trial possible.
- Customised education and training plans will likely be required for the vendors, investigators, and other personnel involved in the trial. Critical thinking is needed from the personnel involved to create flexible technology systems and procedures required to execute these clinical trials.
- During the conduct, it is important to document what happened, maintain a proper firewall, and manage external communications effectively. For long-term platform trials, study adjustments may be unavoidable, but it is important that these adjustments are made before the patients are enrolled into the new study arm.

Introduction

There is no one best design, method, or approach to clinical trial research. It is not wise to use conventional trial designs by default, nor is it a good idea to always force adaptive trial designs into clinical questions [1]. The same can be said for basket, umbrella, and platform trials. Basket trials and umbrella trials can be useful in identifying disease-agnostic targeted therapies or those targeting biomarker sub-types, but the precision medicine approach is not always applicable nor is it useful [2]. Making the business case for platform trials is easy in fields with multiple competing therapies or in rare diseases in which patient recruitment is difficult or not possible without extensive collaboration, but this is not always the case [3]. Any absolute statement or endorsement towards one specific approach should be avoided.

We feel comfortable stating that the criteria for good clinical trial research starts with asking an important research question and then answering it reliably, and research methods are merely tools for clinical trial research [4]. There will be benefits associated with adopting adaptive trial designs and master protocols, but they should be carefully weighed against risks and anticipated challenges. This is not to deter the use of adaptive trial designs and master protocols. Taking on these challenges for adaptive trial designs and master protocols is generally well worth the effort with proper planning and resourcing. However, different design choices will have their trade-offs, since the expected performance of each design will vary between scenarios and different assumptions.

In this chapter, we discuss practical considerations for clinical trial planning and execution for complex clinical trials in those adaptive, basket, umbrella, and platform trial designs. For further discussion on practical considerations of adaptive trial designs, the readers can also refer to PANDAS (A Practical Adaptive & Novel Designs and Analysis) toolkit (https://panda.shef.ac.uk/). We assume that there is a strong scientific rationale already established for the purpose of our discussion. Herein, we have structured our discussion into the planning (statistical design and operational planning) and execution stages of adaptive trial designs and master protocols, followed by a discussion of funding. The actual process of clinical trial research may be more of a continuum and highly iterative, especially for basket, umbrella, and platform trials since they may involve multiple sub-studies. Statistical considerations are important, but they are only the half the picture. In addition to having desirable operating characteristics, it is important to ensure that all specified trial design requirements can be executed as intended. The planned adaptations, once triggered, need to be implemented as seamlessly as possible without creating potential operational bias. Our experience tells us that additional time and resources for planning are often required for adaptive, basket, umbrella, and platform trials. Cross-functional coordination will be required up front between clinical trialists, statisticians, research coordinators, data managers, and many others with expertise in operational planning and execution.

Planning Considerations

Requirements for Adaptive Trial Designs

Adaptive clinical trials require the data being used to guide adaptations to be collected, entered, and analysed in a timely fashion. The measurement of the primary endpoint should be sufficiently quick relative to the anticipated recruitment for the interim analyses to result in a meaningful change before the trial is completed. It is possible to recruit in stages with paused enrolment in between, but this could lengthen the overall duration of the trial. In addition, from an operational standpoint it is typically best to avoid pausing enrolment, as it can make it very difficult to enrol patients. It is also possible to consider using a surrogate endpoint that can be measure more quickly, given that treatment effect measured by a surrogate endpoint is able to predict the treatment effect on the true endpoint; however, this is not always easy to determine [5]. It is recommended to consult with regulatory agencies and other key stakeholders early to assess the acceptability of the surrogate endpoint.

Design Planning

Governance Structure

It is important to establish an effective governance structure early since the planning and execution of complex clinical trials will require a keen oversight. There should be appropriate representations from all stakeholders, and they should be provided with decision-making authority to ensure that the trial can function with an effective oversight. There is usually one central group that will provide overall accountability, oversight, and responsibility. They will often secure resources and funding to lead the development of the proposal and then the trial design. It is often the case that there are multiple companies contributing their therapeutic interventions to be evaluated in basket, umbrella, and platform trials [6, 7]. The members of the central group making the overall strategic and executive direction of these trials should ideally be without conflict.

It is critical to identify statistical experts early and engage them extensively throughout to establish critical research questions and estimands to inform the protocol design. They will be required to perform the simulations and to develop the statistical analysis plan. Statisticians can continue to function as part of the central group, or they can come from the independent statistical analysis centre to carry out the unblinded statistical analyses. Once the trial starts and data are being analysed, these statisticians should function independently from the central group. The plans to support the data monitoring activities of the independent Data and Safety Monitoring Board (DSMB) should be discussed and outlined in the terms of reference and other governance documents.

The independence of the DSMB is important to maintain their objectivity throughout the conduct of the trial [8]. Their independence, however, should not be confused with freedom for these members to change the trial design as they see fit. Their roles and responsibilities should be clearly outlined in their DSMB charter with information on the planned adaptations and statistical design [8]. The core function of the DSMB is to ensure patient safety with a secondary function to protect the trial integrity. They will require access to full unblinded trial data to accurately determine the risk-benefit ratio of the treatments being evaluated in the trial. Their role is not to re-design the trial and make stopping decisions for efficacy without pre-specified stopping rules. They cannot stop the trial for efficacy on their own, so there are limited concerns around inflating the type I error rate with the DSMB having access to unblinded efficacy data. The DSMB can recommend the trial stop for patient protection in case of safety concerns to protect the patients.

In platform trials, it is common for the governance structure to include therapeutic sub-committees or leads that are responsible for the design and oversight of the specific therapies. They will raise issues and key items of the treatment to the central group. To guide the decision-making process on what and when new interventions will be added, having a Research Prioritisation Committee that can review the scientific merits of new interventions being considered in accordance with the established prioritization criteria is also helpful [9, 10]. The governance structure should be determined on a case-by-case basis, but terms of reference outlining their composition, communication path, and responsibilities should be clearly outlined a priori before the trial starts.

Structure of the Master Protocol

The protocol structure deserves consideration to ensure that protocol amendments (e.g., new arms being added and or arms being dropped) can be made more seamlessly in platform trials, as well as basket and umbrella trials, if they are designed to add new sub-studies over time. In anticipation of multiple amendments, it is important to plan for clear version control measures that can ensure that different trial sites and their staff can easily identify the active version of the protocol documents [11].

There are many ways in which a master protocol can be structured. Two main ways include single versus modular protocol structures. The single protocol document is the most common way in which clinical trials are organised. Here, there is a single protocol document that contains all information about the trial. The details on administrative information; background, rationale, trial objectives of the trial; eligibility criteria; interventions; outcomes; schedule of activities; recruitment; randomisation and blinding methods; data collection, management, and analysis; monitoring; statistical design; and other information would be outlined in one document [12].

Under the modular structure, there would be a core master protocol document that would contain common generic elements and information of the trial including the documented standardised operating procedures. Specific information ön the sub-studies and their specific interventions could be outlined in sub-protocol or other documents as appendices. There could be intervention-specific appendices that outline intervention-specific protocol elements. There can also be other non-interventional appendix documents outlining other design details, such as a statistical analysis plan (SAP) and simulation appendices that contain a pre-specified statistical analysis plan, adaptations, and the simulated trial operating characteristics [13].

Adopting a singular protocol structure does make it easier to track the active version of the protocol. This can make amendments less seamless, since when an intervention is added or discontinued, the entire protocol document needs to be updated. The main benefit of adopting a modular structure includes the possibility of expediting the process of adding new interventions, since the core master protocol does not need to be updated every time there is a change to the trial. When a new intervention is added, a new intervention-specific appendix can be added. Administrative requirements such as an institutional ethical review could be expedited, as the trial design for the new intervention is typically identical to the design that was first approved. New interventions may then be indicated in an amendment to the trial protocol rather than requiring a completely new review [14]. However, adopting a modular structure can raise other administrative challenges. Based on our experience, site-level research coordinators have reported challenges in keeping track of the active versions of the protocol across the multiple documents. There are no right or wrong answers to how the master protocol should be structured. The structure should be determined on case-by-case basis.

Simulation-Guided Trial Design

Using clinical trial simulation as a guide for trial planning (simulation-guided trial design) is generally beneficial regardless of the designs being considered [15]. In conventional trial designs and less complicated adaptive trial designs, such as classical group sequential designs, the operating characteristics can be derived analytically without simulations. For complex trials, simulations are required to demonstrate the control of the type I error rate across multiple null effect scenarios [16–18]. In either case, it is still beneficial to use clinical trial simulation, since it allows for a detailed risk-benefit analysis of the design under plausible scenarios with different assumptions. Clinical trial simulation can be used to compare multiple design candidates to decide on the highly efficient trial design for the research question being considered.

It is critical that the process of simulation-guided trial design planning involve more than just statisticians [19]. There should be an integrated team with expertise in content, regulatory affairs, clinical operations, and more. Guided by the statisticians, content and other experts will need to come up with a range of plausible scenarios to explore and to examine the operating characteristics of the competing designs [19]. In addition to the statistical considerations, simulations can be used to test for the operational feasibility of the designs including the potential adaptations that are being considered. Recruitment rate, time required to obtain study approval, data cleaning and interim analysis, drug supply, resource allocations, and other operational assumptions can be used to test whether the trial design can actually be executed [20]. Such simulation of operational assessment can help modify the study design to improve its feasibility and be used for logistics planning including drug supply management.

When planning adaptive trial designs, the timing and frequency of interim analyses are critical considerations. There is often conflict between planning analyses early enough to have meaningful benefits for the trial versus balancing the loss of information (i.e., having less data) on the experimental treatments and control [21]. Planning the interim analyses too late will result in negligible benefits for the trial, but this should be balanced with the trial being designed to allow for sufficient data to be collected. More frequent interim analyses will increase the expected statistical efficiency as well as the operational demands. It is important to recognise that sequential designs by design are used to deliver less information [21]. Even with valid statistical measures to control for false positive error and minimal loss in statistical power, there is no escaping that statistical inference may be based on less data [21]. Most adaptive trial designs use a single endpoint to guide the adaptations, so optimising the trial design too aggressively can make secondary analyses on secondary efficacy endpoints, sub-groups, and safety much more challenging.

When planning interim analyses, there needs to be a decision made on what data will be included in the interim analysis and what happens after a decision is made in the case of sequential designs. For instance, while waiting for the results of the interim analysis, there extra data can be collected, a phenomenon that is referred to as overrunning [22, 23]. There may be patients already enrolled finishing up their clinical follow-up, or new patients may be enrolled into the trial during the waiting time. If decision to stop the study arm is made based on the interim analysis, it is important to recognise that the results may change after the analysis is updated with the additional 'overrun' data. The a priori decision should be made explicitly to determine whether the study arm (or the trial in the case of a two-arm trial) should stop early based on the data available at the interim analysis or based on the updated analysis with all data that are collected in the trial. It is possible to pause enrolment at the time of the interim analysis and make the final decision based on the most complete data. This may not be ideal, but making the final decision on the most complete data may be preferable.

Operational Planning

Vendor and Site Selection

The vendors should be involved in the trial as soon as possible, preferably at the design stage. The plans for the key events between different stages of the trial should be outlined with details for the operational process and personnel that will be involved prior to the start of the trial. Measures to implement adaptations blindly to the site and the sponsor should be discussed to prevent operational bias.

Despite the growing adoption of adaptive, basket, umbrella, and platform clinical trials, it not uncommon for vendors, trial sites, and investigators to lack experience in participating in these complex clinical trials. Clinical trials using an adaptive trial design require high-quality data to be readily available to support the frequent interim analyses to manage their accelerated pace. Clinical trials using a master protocol framework often involve multiple sub-studies, so there are increased demands on trial sites. Trial sites require adequate training and support to handle the requirements of fast data entry, effective drug management and accountability, coordination with vendors for data processing and cleaning, and other aspects of trial management [20].

In an ideal world, we can select qualified vendors, sites, and investigators with proven track records of successfully executing these clinical trials. This is not often the luxury for the clinical trialists. Not all adaptive, basket, umbrella, and platform trials are created equally, so inexperienced sites and investigators may not be at a disadvantage, especially if they are provided with proper education and training. Once the design has been planned more concretely, it is a good idea to think of developing customised training resources that can help build capacity for the specific needs of the trial. It is critical that the investigators are all on the same page with an understanding of the operational demands to successfully execute the trial design as intended.

Common Screening Platform

Establishing a common screening platform is critical for basket, umbrella, and platform trials that operate under a common master protocol. For these trials using a master protocol framework, there are usually two levels of eligibility criteria. First, there are common eligibility criteria at the level of the core protocol, and more specific eligibility criteria are applied at the sub-study or intervention level. In basket, umbrella, and other trials that are biomarker-guided, high screening failures may be unavoidable if the biomarker target is relatively rare [2]. It is vital for the success of these complex trials that there are measures to minimise screening failures and to streamline the recruitment process in a coordinated fashion [7].

Electronic Data Capture System

An electronic data capture (EDC) system is vital for all clinical trials. The careful design and testing of electronic case report forms (eCRFs) are crucial to ensure that essential data elements across all patients and their scheduled visits can be reliably collected. If the interim data contain a large degree of errors, this will be detrimental for the conduct of the adaptive trial. There should be measures in place to ensure quality data collection and timely data entry. The procedures for data processing and transfer should be discussed and planned to support timely interim analyses. Before the trial starts, a decision needs to be made about what data will be included in the interim analyses. It is not always necessary to ensure that all data be collected and processed for interim analyses, since the statistical criteria for the planned decision rules can be calculated using only a few data variables. The eCRFs and EDC system should be user tested and validated before the trial starts.

Randomisation

The randomisation list is predetermined prior to the start of the trial with treatment supplies that are linked being sent to the site. It is often the case that the investigator will log into an interactive web response system (IWRS) or call into an interactive voice response system (IVRS) to randomised patients, after which they will identify the treatment supplies that will need to be either administered or provided to the patient. The database created for the trial will often be linked to the randomisation system to ensure that patients who pass the screening the process can be more readily randomised and recruited into the trial. It is possible to randomise patients using manual randomisation, but this is very rare, since complex clinical trials often require complex and flexible randomisation systems.

There are several randomisation challenges with adaptive and other complex trials. The most common randomisation technique that ends up being used is stratified permuted block randomisation with trial sites being used as a stratum [24]. Multiple sites are usually required to allow for a timely recruitment. In open-label trials, the use of block randomisation can make the allocation more predictable. It may be wise to consider less predictable allocation procedures [25]. It might be beneficial to package drug supplies in a different ratio than the planned allocation ratio to make it less predictable.

Most technology systems, including the randomisation system, are designed to carry out conventional trial designs. When there is a decision made to stop enrolment to a study arm, it is important that the randomisation system can seamlessly limit further allocation to that arm. In platform trials in which new study arms can be added, the randomisation system will need to be able to accommodate such change. Response adaptive randomisation will require complex randomisation systems that might be more costly. Such budget considerations should be part of the planning process when weighing the merits of different design types.

Study Approval Planning

Early engagement with the regulatory agency is important to discuss and resolve any issues related to the clinical trial design and execution plans and incorporate their feedback. This is especially important for registrational clinical trials before submitting clinical trial applications for approval. The statistical details of these complex trials can be challenging, so adaptive trial designs and master protocols will often be required to explain these details to an ethics review board. Obtaining study approval may take longer, so this should be considered in the planning stage. For platform trials, adding a new arm will be expedited if this amendment can be considered as a minor amendment by the ethics review board. However, since not many ethics review boards have experience running platform trials, they may still require a full review, even if the only change being made to the trial is addition of the new intervention.

Execution Considerations

Documentation

Regardless of the trial design used, proper documentation is required to ensure that the established processes were properly adhered to. Proper documentation should enable an independent observer to reconfirm the data and events that occurred throughout the conduct [26]. Documentation should provide an audit trail to permit investigation, if and when one is required [26]. The principle of 'if it wasn't recorded, it never happened' should be followed as a rule.

Firewall

To minimise operational bias, trial information needs to be tightly controlled. Interim analyses should be performed by the independent statistical centre and reviewed by the independent DSMB. Appropriate firewalls and processes should be in place to ensure that access to the trial results is restricted to the right personnel only and to prevent information leakage that may impact the integrity of the trial [27]. For instance, it is acceptable for the trial investigators to attend the open session of the DSMB meetings to ensure that the DSMB is fully informed of the study design and what it is being asked to guide. Communications with the DSMB should not convey any information about the comparative effectiveness results until there are concerns for safety or other ethical issues, or until the DSMB is prepared to make a major recommendation in accordance with the pre-specified plans.

Interim analyses and knowledge of the executed adaptations can reveal some information about the treatment effects of the ongoing intervention. In the case of sample size re-estimation design, knowing that the trial increased the sample size target can reveal information of the treatment effect. Similar issues may arise in the case of response adaptive randomisation if the allocation numbers are revealed. This could be problematic, especially in open-label studies. Strict communication and information flow structure will need to be maintained with the independent statistical analysis centre and the DSMB.

External Communications

For platform trials or other long-term trials, the potential for information leakage may be unavoidable but should be minimised as much as possible. The data from ongoing interventions or a shared control group will be revealed when platform trial results of an intervention that finished evaluation are made public in forms of conference presentations and peer-reviewed publications. It is not always clear how the results should be reported for an intervention arm that was found to be more effective than the control group for a specific patient sub-type (e.g., biomarker sub-type) when it is still being evaluated in other patient groups. If the same intervention is still being evaluated in other remaining groups, scientific communication may be delayed until the intervention is no longer active to preserve trial integrity. It may be important for the central group to determine the amount of information that can be publicly shared. It is our opinion that any results of an intervention that is still being evaluated in the trial should be delayed for publications.

Making Adjustments Mid-Trial

In the case of platform trials, adjustments to the statistical analysis plan and other aspects of the trial design are often necessary, given its long-term nature. A new estimand may be proposed when a new intervention to be added into the trial is being considered [28]. Since this may require a different estimator (statistical analysis plan), this will likely require new simulations to be conducted. In such a case, the details on the analysis plan should be finalised before patients start being randomised to the new treatment arm. There can be other instances in which simulations are required to fine-tune the statistical design of ongoing platform trials. For instance, throughout the conduct of the TOGETHER trial, as we knew the hospitalisation rates rapidly declined due to more vaccines becoming widely available, simulations were conducted to adjust the statistical design and sample size target before new treatment arms were added. The statistical design team of the TOGETHER trial were blinded and independent of the statistical analysis centre, so there were limited concerns.

Funding Considerations

The public funding model is typically designed to support conventional clinical trials. It is unfortunate, but the academic funding process is not designed to enable more adaptive trial designs and master protocols to be conducted. In public funding models, single-agent or per-project-based grant funding is usually awarded. Public funding is structured mostly to test a single, or perhaps numerous, intervention. Even though different research questions may vary considerably in scope, the funding amount is usually fixed for most grant applications. For example, in the case of sample size re-estimation design, it is unlikely for public funders to increase the funding amount when there is a promising signal of the treatment effect that warrants increasing the sample size. Similarly, public funders do not typically support the long-term infrastructure for clinical trials without planning what the intended interventions may be. Drug developers, on the other hand, may benefit from findings at interim analyses, as they can use the news of promising interim results to raise additional finances [29, 30]. However, public granting agencies are currently not structured this way.

Based on our experience, obtaining predictable long-term funding is the biggest challenge, even more so than some of the statistical design and implementation challenges discussed above. Obtaining multiple funding sources is difficult but often required, especially in the case of platform trials that are designed to be perpetual or at least very long term. Philanthropic organisations have played an important role in funding some of these complex platform trials for COVID-19. The Wellcome Trust, Unitaid, Bill & Melinda Gates Foundation, Fast Grants, and FTX Foundation are examples of agencies that have supported platform trials. In other instances, some trials have specifically formulated a separate fund-raising committee to financially support the ongoing trial [31]. The pay-to-play model in which different industry partners contribute per-patient cost to the ongoing trial has worked for several platform trials [31].

Conclusion

This chapter is intended as a high-level overview of the different considerations that are required to come up with clinical trial designs and execute them. The planning and execution are complex and involve coordination and partnership with many groups. There are several processes that will need to be linked through common systems. Running clinical trials, especially those with more complex trial designs, are certainly not easy. This is not to deter the use of adaptive trial designs and master protocol frameworks. When considering these complex trials, it is important to ask whether the possible benefits outweigh the extra efforts required to implement the planned design. Using clinical trial simulation helps to weigh the pros and cons to make the final decision in a formal analytical framework. The other practical considerations covered in this chapter will be important for trial planning. Based on our experience, they are fun challenges and worth the extra effort. Proper planning does take time, so please do plan in advance.

References

1. Wason JM, Brocklehurst P, Yap C. When to keep it simple – adaptive designs are not always useful. *BMC Med.* 2019;17(1):1–7.

2. Antoniou M, Kolamunnage-Dona R, Wason J, et al. Biomarker-guided trials: challenges in practice. *Contemp Clin Trials Commun.* 2019;16:100493.

3. Lee KM, Wason J, Stallard N. To add or not to add a new treatment arm to a multiarm study: a decision-theoretic framework. *Stat Med.* 2019;38(18):3305–21.

4. Yusuf S, Collins R, Peto R. Why do we need some large, simple randomized trials? *Stat Med.* 1984;3(4):409–20.

5. Krendyukov A, Singhvi S, Zabransky M. Value of adaptive trials and surrogate endpoints for clinical decision-making in rare cancers. *Front Oncol.* 2021;**11**:636561.

6. Park JJH, Siden E, Zoratti MJ, et al. Systematic review of basket trials, umbrella trials, and platform trials: a landscape analysis of master protocols. *Trials.* 2019;**20**(1):572.

7. Woodcock J, LaVange LM. Master protocols to study multiple therapies, multiple diseases, or both. *N Eng J Medicine.* 2017;**377**(1):62–70.

8. DAMOCLES Study Group. A proposed charter for clinical trial data monitoring committees: helping them to do their job well. *Lancet.* 2005;**365**(9460):711–22.

9. Barker AD, Sigman CC, Kelloff GJ, et al. I-SPY 2: an adaptive breast cancer trial design in the setting of neoadjuvant chemotherapy. *Clin Pharmacol Ther.* 2009;**86**(1):97–100.

10. Sydes MR, Parmar MK, James ND, et al. Issues in applying multi-arm multi-stage methodology to a clinical trial in prostate cancer: the MRC STAMPEDE trial. *Trials.* 2009;**10**:39.

11. Hague D, Townsend S, Masters L, et al. Changing platforms without stopping the train: experiences of data management and data management systems when adapting platform protocols by adding and closing comparisons. *Trials.* 2019;**20**(1):294.

12. Chan AW, Tetzlaff JM, Altman DG, et al. SPIRIT 2013 statement: defining standard protocol items for clinical trials. *Ann Intern Med.* 2013;**158**(3):200–207.

13. Angus DC, Alexander BM, Berry S, et al. Adaptive platform trials: definition, design, conduct and reporting considerations. *Nat Rev Drug Discov* 2019;**18**(10):797–807.

14. Schiavone F, Bathia R, Letchemanan K, et al. This is a platform alteration: a trial management perspective on the operational aspects of adaptive and platform and umbrella protocols. *Trials.* 2019;**20**(1):264.

15. Mayer C, Perevozskaya I, Leonov S, et al. Simulation practices for adaptive trial designs in drug and device development. *Stat Biopharm Res.* 2019;**11**(4):325–35.

16. United States Department of Health and Human Services, Food and Drug Administration. *Master Protocols: Efficient Clinical Trial Design Strategies to Expedite Development of Oncology Drugs and Biologics Guidance for Industry.* United States Department of Health and Human Services; 2022. www.fda.gov/media/ 120721/download

17. United States Department of Health and Human Services, Food and Drug Administration. *Adaptive Designs for Clinical Trials of Drugs and Biologics. Guidance for Industry.* Center for Biologics Evaluation and Research (CBER); 2019.

18. U.S. Food and Drug Administration. *Adaptive Designs for Medical Device Clinical Studies Guidance for Industry and Food and Drug Administration Staff.* United States Department of Health and Human Services; 2016.

19. Thorlund K, Haggstrom J, Park JJ, Mills EJ. Key design considerations for adaptive clinical trials: a primer for clinicians. *BMJ.* 2018;**360**:k698.

20. Marchenko O, Nolan C. Implementing adaptive designs: operational considerations, putting it all together. In He W, Pinheiro J, Kuznetsova OM, editors. *Practical Considerations for Adaptive Trial Design and Implementation*, pp. 203–23. Springer; 2014.

21. Senn S. Being efficient about efficacy estimation. *Stat Biopharm Res.* 2013;**5** (3):204–10.

22. Baldi I, Azzolina D, Soriani N, et al. Overrunning in clinical trials: some thoughts from a methodological review. *Trials.* 2020;**21**(1):668.

23. Whitehead J. Overrunning and underrunning in sequential clinical trials. *Control Clin Trials.* 1992;**13**(2):106–21.

24. Broglio K. Randomization in clinical trials: permuted blocks and stratification. *JAMA.* 2018;**319**(21):2223–4.

25. Kuznetsova OM. Randomization challenges in adaptive design studies.

In He W, Pinheiro J, Kuznetsova OM, editors. *Practical Considerations for Adaptive Trial Design and Implementation*, pp. 157–81. Springer; 2014.

26. Bargaje C. Good documentation practice in clinical research. *Perspect Clin Res.* 2011;**2** (2):59–63.

27. Detry MA, Lewis RJ, Broglio KR, et al. *Standards for the Design, Conduct, and Evaluation of Adaptive Randomized Clinical Trials.* Patient-Centered Outcomes Research Institute (PCORI); 2012.

28. Collignon O, Schiel A, Burman CF, et al. Estimands and complex innovative designs. *Clin Pharmacol Ther.* 2022. Online ahead of print.

29. Posch M, Bauer P. Adaptive budgets in clinical trials. *Stat Biopharm Res.* 2013;**5** (4):282–92.

30. Ravandi F, Ritchie EK, Sayar H, et al. Vosaroxin plus cytarabine versus placebo plus cytarabine in patients with first relapsed or refractory acute myeloid leukaemia (VALOR): a randomised, controlled, double-blind, multinational, phase 3 study. *Lancet Oncol.* 2015;**16** (9):1025–36.

31. Angus DC, Alexander BM, Berry S, et al. Adaptive platform trials: definition, design, conduct and reporting considerations. *Nat Rev Drug Discov.* 2019;**18**(10):797–808.

Index